BY TERRANCE J. SPAHL, DDS

The Clinical Management of Basic Maxillofacial Orthopedic Appliances, Volume I: Mechanics

The Clinical Management of Basic Maxillofacial Orthopedic Appliances, Volume II: Diagnostics

The Clinical Management of Basic Maxillofacial Orthopedic Appliances, Volume III: Temporomandibular Joint

The Clinical Management of the FJO/TMD/Migraine Continuum: An Evidence-Based Construct

The Headache-Free Wonders of Functional Orthodontics

THE HEADACHE-FREE **WONDERS** OF *FUNCTIONAL* ORTHODONTICS

THE HEADACHE-FREE WONDERS OF FUNCTIONAL ORTHODONTICS

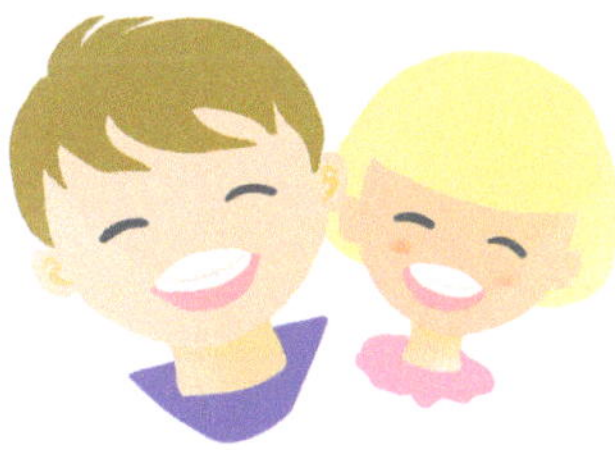

Or

A Concerned Parent's Guide:
How to Choose Proper Orthodontic Care
for Your Child or Yourself

BY DR. T. J. SPAHL

SPAHL DENTISTRY
1199 DULUTH STREET - ST. PAUL, MN

Spahl Dentistry
1199 Duluth St.
St. Paul, MN 55106-2702

in conjunction with

Fire's Edge Publishing
310 N. Derby Lane PO Box 800
North Sioux City, SD 57049

First Edition: April 2021

ISBN 978-1-7349697-0-2 (paperback)
ISBN 978-1-7349697-2-6 (e-book)
Library of Congress Control Number: 2020910075

Editing & Project Management by Cory Kruse
Typesetting & Interior Book Design by Anamaria Stefan
Proofreading by Barry Lyons & Barbara Noe Kennedy

Cover Design by Applefresh

To learn more, visit tjspahldds.com

Printed in the United States of America

To my gracious and loving wife

Susan

The main brace of the Spahl household

CONTENTS

To sin by silence, when we should protest,
makes cowards out of men.

— Ella Wheeler Wilcox (1850–1919),
Excerpt from "Protest"

Introduction

Brace Yourself!

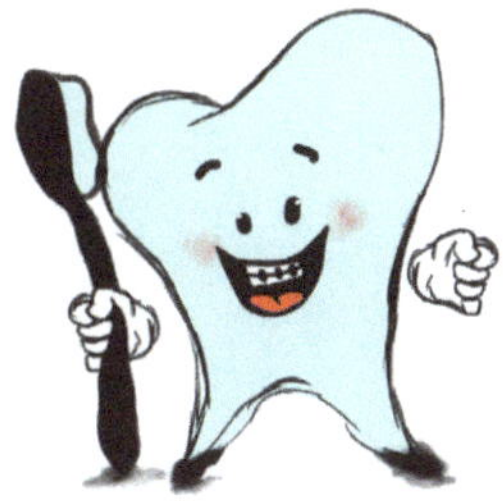

Life being very short, and the quiet hours of it few,
we ought to waste none of them in reading valueless books.

— John Ruskin (1819–1900)
English art critic

I ask you, dear reader, to imagine the scene:

There you sit, sipping your morning coffee and casually perusing the Sunday paper. You pause for a moment to look across the kitchen table at your child—the light of your life and the apple of your eye—busily munching on breakfast flakes while deeply engrossed in the subject matter on the back of the cereal box. You speak your child's name; your adorable offspring looks up at you and smiles. What do you see? A bright, shining, well-scrubbed face accompanied by two sparkling eyes and an unruly yet endearing mop top. But the longer you look, the more your heart sinks because you realize, disconcertedly, that right in the middle of all that beaming sunshine is an irregular gap-toothed grin, one that could qualify as the first runner-up in a Halloween pumpkin-carving contest. Alas, the truth dawns on you: It's time for braces.

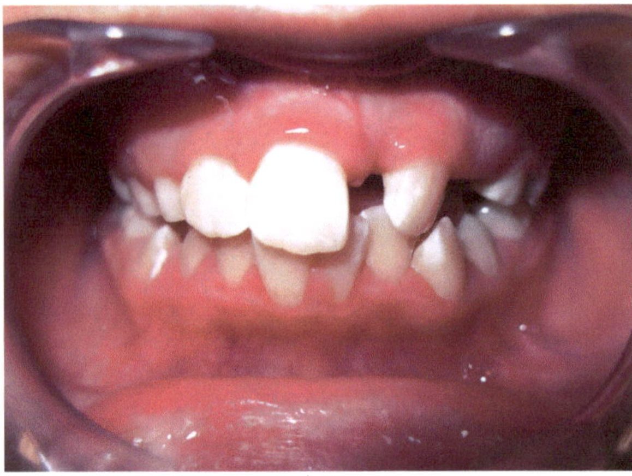

(A)

→ Figure I-A: Yup; it's time for braces.

A quick phone call and a nervous visit to your family dentist later, and you're informed that the problem isn't an easy fix. A few months of treatment with some simple braces or a removable retainer won't do the trick; in this case, a major job involving the services of a specialist is needed. Your family dentist (or maybe the neighbor across the street) makes a recommendation as to whom to see.

So you make another appointment, this time with an orthodontic specialist. After a brief consultation, you're informed that the treatment required will take two to three years, will not be cheap, and four of your child's permanent adult teeth may even have to be removed. This of course not only engenders a deep sense of genetic guilt—as well as a severe sense of fear in your child—but it also requires a referral to yet another dental specialist. This time you visit an *oral surgeon* (a dentist who specializes in extracting teeth), who first puts your child "to sleep" with a combination of gas (nitrous oxide) and, sometimes, even *intravenous anesthesia*. The surgeon then removes the teeth deemed expendable by the orthodontist and sends your child home with a swollen mouth chock-full of cotton gauze, so that the resemblance to a pocket gopher smuggling marshmallows from a summer picnic is unavoidable.

With four teeth now missing at the corners of your child's mouth, the gap-toothed grin is seemingly magnified tenfold until the day when the braces are applied. Your child—totally self-conscious by now—leaves the orthodontist's office with the newly applied metal braces, the dental devices looking as if they could double as some sort of radar apparatus, capable of receiving radio signals from outer space.

If it's your son, he'll probably put the new oral apparatus to the test in his first ice hockey game; if it's your daughter, she'll probably confine herself to her room for a week. Either way, soon their sensitive adolescent egos—and the insides of their mouths—will adapt to all the steel wire and metal hardware, and, after several years of yet more orthodontist visits and innumerable alterations (manipulations, tightenings, and the adjustment of rubber bands, wires, or even the ever-attractive headgear straps), the big day finally—*finally*—comes, and the braces are at last removed.

The ugly duckling has turned into a swan. Your son or daughter's smile seems, at first, as beautiful as any belonging to Brad Pitt or Angelina Jolie. And, to top it all off, the whole thing is even finally paid for.

All parties concerned are satisfied, happy to be finished. At last, it's all over.

Or is it?

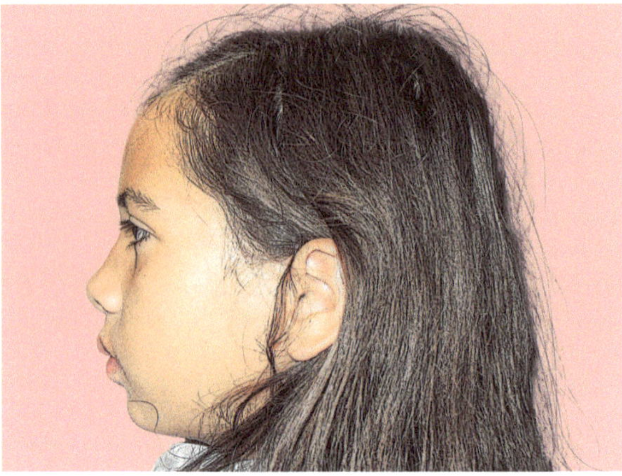

(B)

→ Figure I-B: Not only does the little girl's teeth in Fig. I-1 need a bit of help, but her jaws could use some work, too. Notice the retruded profile of the lower jaw and chin. Additionally, her pre-treatment X-rays portend trouble in the future (we'll explain why in subsequent chapters).

From what we now know, it isn't always so simple. More appointments, more braces, and, to the detriment of your wallet, more expenses might lie ahead. These additional difficulties are often due to the long-term effects of the particular type of orthodontic care that was selected and delivered at the start. Unlike the "old days," modern times present a more nuanced selection, as the proper treatment option is not always as automatic as it used to be. Thus, as a hapless parent, you are once again tasked with making a judgment call concerning your child's welfare—a crossroads of significant consequences. Young Prince Hamlet was right: Life always seems to be filled with tough choices.

Personally, I don't think selecting the proper orthodontic treatment for your child should have to be one of them. Which is why I wrote this book. Between its covers, you'll find the information and resources you need to choose the right treatment option for your child (or yourself), all of it condensed and spelled out in simple "laymen's terms" to help you more easily navigate the complex landscape of orthodontic care. Consider it a helpful little guide for your journey.

That said, I implore you to "brace yourself" for the pages ahead and for the knowledge you'll find there, as you will soon discover that, even in these modern times, a person can't always depend on the professionals to make the right decision. Wonderful new techniques have emerged in the "tooth-straightening business," techniques that many patients—as well as their dental clinicians—will greatly benefit from. But dental professionals don't always employ such treatment options, whether out of simple ignorance or due to a proclivity for old methods. And therein lies the problem.

The world at large is witnessing a new era in orthodontic care, spurred on by a monumental series of technical revolutions that have made orthodontics (and its twin sister, the diagnosis and treatment of *cranio-mandibular disorders*) an exciting, rapidly changing field, one that's seen spectacular results including the correction of life-long headaches and even migraines! Nevertheless, these advancements have also generated a certain amount of controversy. Because these breakthroughs are relatively new, and are often viewed as too dramatic or progressive, they can sometimes catch dental practitioners off guard.

As a result, some orthodontic patients get caught in the academic crossfire—and fail to receive the treatment they need.

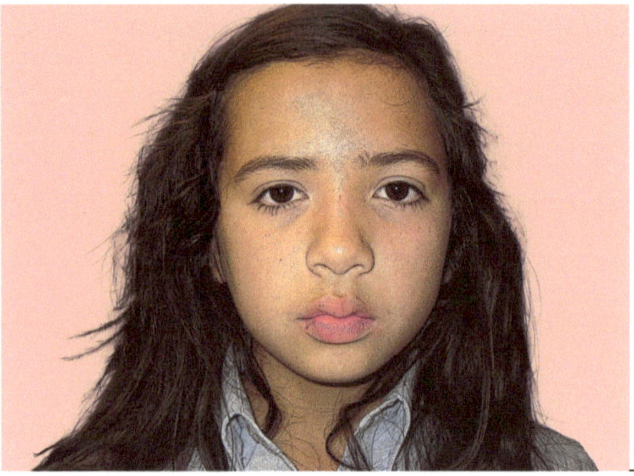

(C)

→ Figure I-C: As you can see, the patient is now reluctant to smile.

Such an impasse affects millions of patients every year; many have no choice but to deal with the lasting consequences. Yet hope remains! A growing number of clinicians, academics, and trailblazers from across the orthodontic field are pressing onward, praising these advanced methods "to the hilt" and, for the sake of *all* patients, are endeavoring to promote their widespread use.

Over time, because of the efforts of these intrepid professionals, the field of orthodontics will continue to evolve. Let's take a look at why that's so important—and what it means for you.

ONE

Dental Nomenclature for Newbies

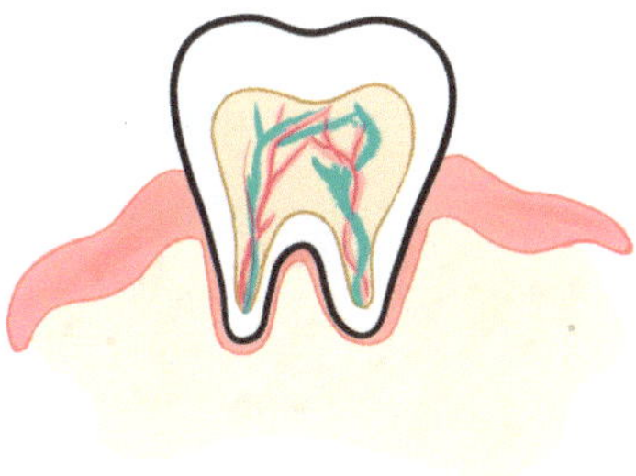

Man with all his noble qualities ... still bears in his bodily frame the indelible stamp of his lowly origin.

— Charles Darwin (1809–1882),
English naturalist

Don't be insulted.

I know you're not a so-called "newbie." However, unless you have an extensive biological background at the collegiate level, a dissertation on a subject as complicated as orthodontics would be near impossible to understand without first learning a bit of basic biological, anatomical, and scientific language.

It isn't a language that's hard to learn—and for our purposes here in this little book, there won't be much anyhow—so I believe you'll quickly get the hang of it. In the spirit of that popular series of large yellow paperbacks, which aims to make complicated subjects accessible to the uninitiated layperson, let's take a very brief and relaxed sojourn through just a few of the scientific dental terms we will need for the remainder of this text. (If you do in fact have some sort of dental/medical background, or feel you already possess a solid grasp of the following terms and concepts, give yourself five extra-credit points and proceed immediately to the next chapter. For everyone else, go someplace quiet where you can concentrate, grab a snack, and get comfortable. I promise this won't take long. Knowledge is power, and you need to know this.)

The *human adult dentition* is composed of 32 teeth (although it is steadily becoming apparent that the modern human jaws are really only programmed, size-wise, for 28). The *pediatric dentition* (baby or milk teeth, or the *deciduous dentition*) is composed of only 20 teeth, 10 in each upper and lower jaw. All of these are designed to be shed as the jaws grow bigger, each eventually replaced by its own corresponding larger adult tooth. Isn't it nice how that all works out?

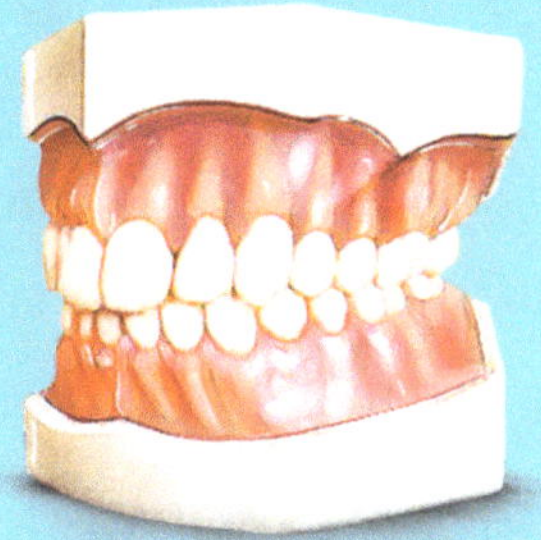

(A)

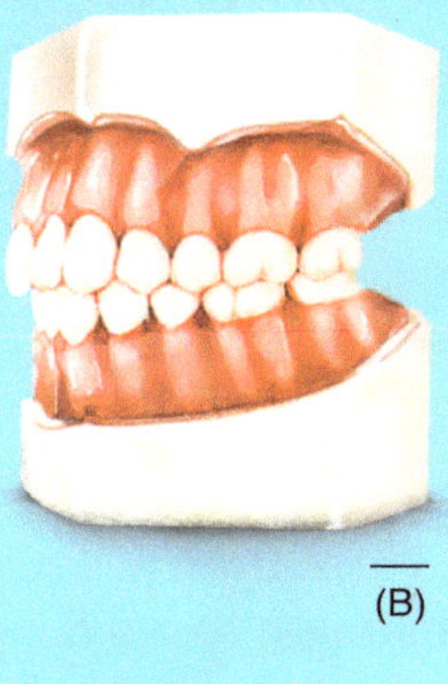

(B)

→ Figure 1-1 (A): Quartering view of a plastic model showing a normal arrangement of teeth at full bite (*occlusion*), the type of bite dentists refer to as *Dental Class I*. Note how nearly three fourths of the facial surfaces of the lower front teeth show at full occlusion, with about only one fourth of the frontal surfaces of these teeth tucked up under the upper front teeth. The amount of vertical overlap at full occlusion is referred to as *vertical dimension of occlusion* (or VDO). Usually, dentists shorten the term and just refer to it as "vertical." When the upper front teeth cover a major portion (or even all) of the lower front teeth, such a condition is called a *deep overbite*.

→ Figure 1-1 (B): Lateral view of the same set of anatomically ideal teeth and fit of the bite. The vertical overlap of the front teeth at full bite is referred to as *overbite*, while the horizontal distance between the biting edges of the upper front teeth out over the tops of the lower front teeth is called *overjet* (like a jet plane taking off horizontally down a runway). Normally, it should be about 1 millimeter or less; i.e., very little.

Teeth

In discussing the human dentition and the jaw mechanisms that make it work, we must look briefly at three key areas: the teeth themselves, the bones in which they reside, and, finally, the muscles that drive and operate the entire jaw apparatus.

A *tooth* is really a highly modified bone. The part that sticks up through the gum tissue is called the *crown*. It is covered with a thick, incredibly hard crystalline capping material called *enamel*. Enamel is dead—like your hair or fingernails—but the main body of the tooth, just underneath the outer layer of enamel, is a living, highly modified bone-like material named *dentin*. Dentin is alive and extremely solid, but not nearly as durable as the outer layer of enamel. The major bodily portion of the tooth lies below the gum line; it's known as the *root structure*. Like the roots of a tree, the roots of teeth spread deep into the jawbones, where they are securely anchored within their sockets. Because the roots are not only hard but are also made out of dentin—and therefore alive—there is a thin, but very tough, little membrane that grows throughout the inner surface of each socket and attaches itself to both the entire root surfaces of the teeth and to the bony socket walls. It is this little sheath of ligament tissue that allows braces to work. But more on that in a moment.

The six large upper teeth across the front of the dental arch—the ones we see when we look at ourselves straight on in the mirror, which are occasionally referred to as "the social six"—are called *upper incisors*.

They do just that: incise or cut through things (such as a crisp, juicy apple). They are matched in the front of the mouth top to bottom, six uppers against six lowers, although the upper incisors are much wider than their lower equivalents. The large pointed teeth at either end of this set of six are called *cuspids* or *canines*. There are four cuspids in total, one at each corner of the dental arches. They are equivalent to the canines of carnivores, which is why they're sometimes referred to by that name. Overall, they are incredibly strong, have huge roots, and are very important.

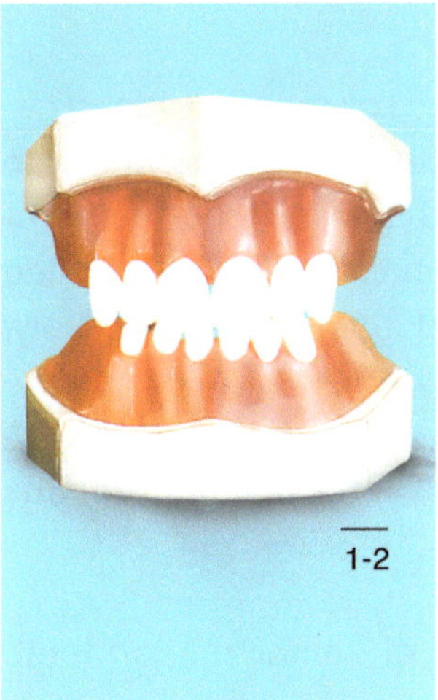

→ Figure 1-2: A view of the upper front and lower front teeth only. Note the overbite/overjet relationships. These teeth are called *anterior incisors*. The uppers are called *maxillary incisors*, or, sometimes, *upper anteriors*. Sometimes, they are nicknamed "the social six" because they're the teeth that show the most when we smile.The lowers are called *mandibular incisors*, or just plain *lower incisors*.

The big grinding teeth way in the back are named *molars*. There are three molars in each of the four rear sections—what we call *quadrants*—of your mouth. The most important of these is the first molar—sometimes described as the *six-year molar*, because it typically shows up (in each of the four quadrants) at about six years of age, right behind the last *deciduous* (or baby) tooth. The first molars don't replace any of the 20 pre-existing baby teeth but merely erupt into the mouth on their own, free and clear. So, by the time we are six years old, we should have 24 teeth in total: the original 20 baby teeth and the four six-year molars.

Right behind these first molars another set of teeth develop: the *second* or *12-year molars*. These teeth begin in the jawbone below the gums but eventually erupt into the mouth—again, one in each quadrant—around the age of 11 or 12 (hence the name). Yet another set develops anywhere between ages 18–25, directly behind the 12-year molars in each quadrant. These are the famous *wisdom teeth* (or, *third molars*). The general purpose of all of these "big brutes" in the back is to grind up food.

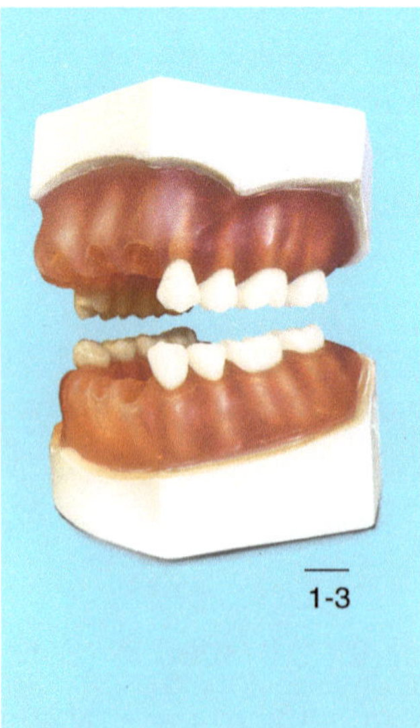

1-3

→ Figure 1-3: A view of the bite with the upper and lower front teeth removed. The remaining teeth are called *premolars* and *molars*. Collectively, they are merely referred to as *posteriors*. In anatomical terminology, *anterior* means "front" and *posterior* means "back."

Note: This set of demonstration teeth and jaws is referred to as a *typodont*; the plastic teeth are removable from their sockets of rubber gums for demonstration and teaching purposes.

Between the six thin, biting incisors in the front of the mouth and the big, sturdy molars way in the back, there are a series of intermediate teeth known as the bicuspids (or, *premolars*). There are four *first bicuspids*; right behind them are their four almost-identical companions, *the second bicuspids*.

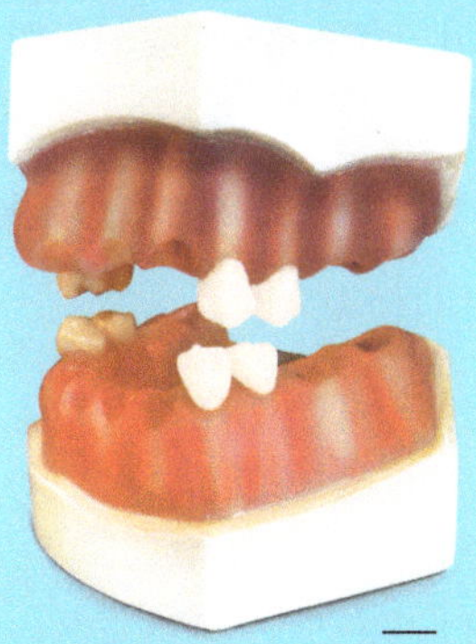
1-4

→ Figure 1-4: In this view, most of the plastic teeth have been removed to show the teeth (two each per quadrant) that are referred to as bicuspids or (a bit more formally) as premolars. These were the teeth often selected in the old days for extraction to make room for the *realignment* (straightening) of the rest as well as to make room for the reduction of the large overjets of upper incisors in some cases of severe "buck teeth." One premolar per quadrant was the normal extraction protocol; there are better methods now, in modern times.

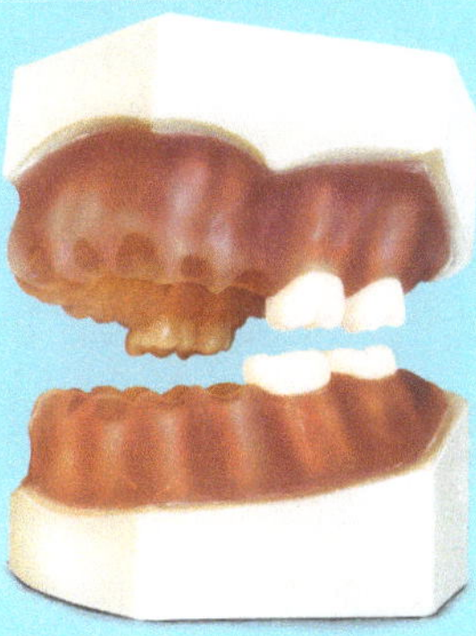
1-5

→ Figure 1-5: The large grinding teeth posterior to the bicuspids are the big molars. In this typodont, the third molars or "wisdom teeth" do not appear. Usually, they are extracted or *impacted* (i.e., stuck down under the bone at the back of the jaws). As a result, they are not often seen in the mouth in proper position. However, in these modern times, certain dentists have figured out clever ways to take advantage of them!

Two bicuspids—a first and a second—sit together in pairs, in each of the four quadrants: upper right, upper left, lower right, and lower left. These teeth are smaller than the big grinding molars and are considered to be only "sort of grinders"—i.e., not as big as the hefty molars in the back, but not as thin and sharp as the front incisors either. They form a graceful dental transition from front to back and are easily seen at the corners of the mouth when we smile broadly. The bicuspids are also the teeth that orthodontists have traditionally deemed expendable in solving some of the perplexing problems of a mouth full of crooked, crowded, jumbled-up teeth. As such, they are often the ones extracted—one out of each quadrant—to make room for the orthodontic realignment of the remaining teeth.

Jaw Muscles

As for the muscles that work the jaws, they have a newfound status in modern orthodontics they never used to enjoy. One main reason for this is we've figured out how to "straighten" them, too!

Now, mind you, there isn't actually such a thing as a crooked jaw muscle; it's just an expression. (Some stuffy members of the dental community get bent out of shape when you use colorful phrases to describe anything scientific.) However, jaw muscles that don't work quite right can seriously deform and/or misalign portions of the highly pliable bones in a set of growing jaws. If you develop crooked (deformed) jawbones, you automatically get a crooked set of teeth. The individual teeth, then, are not the culprits but the victims in the "crooked bite" of a *malocclusion* (mal = "bad," *occlude* = "to close"). They're like innocent passengers on a bus going the wrong direction down a one-way street; they're merely along for the ride. The notion that there could be such a thing as "crooked" jaw muscles—which could deform and/or misalign the upper or lower jawbones, sometimes in very subtle and sneaky ways—was a concept never fully understood by dentists until recently. But now, we can deal with this like never before. This is really big news!

The combined anatomy of the jaw and facial musculature is an elegant, beautiful, artistic, and, alas, very complicated picture. An anatomical drawing of them without any external skin covering is a horrific sight for the layperson, akin to something out of a Stephen King horror movie, so, for now, we will dispense with the image. It is enough for our purposes to merely understand that the jaw muscles themselves are powerful; they come in matched pairs, left and right; and, for all intents and purposes (again, to keep things simple), they are basically divided by function: three pairs to close the jaws, and two pairs to lift them open. Surprisingly, that is all that's needed to work the jaws for chewing.

What's important to note about the jaw muscles used for chewing is that, to a certain extent, they are functionally quite adaptable and are very much creatures of habit. They are also very often the culprits responsible for not only some of the subtle bone deformities that can develop in children, but also the not-so-subtle major deformities and even misalignments of top-to-bottom jaws.

When the individual upper and lower jawbones deform to a significant degree during growth—or even become seriously misaligned, top to bottom, during biting—their "passenger" dentition can ultimately be reflected as a set of crooked teeth. Improperly operating jaw muscles are so powerful that they can sometimes, over the long term, even bring about the partial or complete destruction of the tough, gristled hinge connection that connects the lower jaw joint to the base of the skull, back by the ear (we call this the *temporomandibular joint* [or TMJ]—a big name for such a small joint!). It may be a bit of a stretch, but, if you'll grant me the poetic license to describe it this way for simplicity's sake:

"Crooked" muscles are just as big a player in the development of a poorly fitting or unattractive bite as crooked teeth are—maybe even more so!

But wait, there's more.

Bone

An orthodontic instructor of mine back in dental school once made the comment, "Bone is bone is bone." I can't remember what point he was trying to make (after all, it was more than 50 years ago), but it does bring us to a very important topic that is critical to understanding all of this. Contrary to what some might think, all bone is *not* alike, which is a crucial point in understanding why there is still so much controversy over the new treatment methods in modern orthodontics. In fact, there are three separate categories of bone found in the human body. (Now don't get nervous; we won't be getting very technical. It's just that we will be introducing a few additional terms in order to clarify that very important point.)

The first type of bone in the human body is called c*hondral bone* (from the scientific word for "cartilage"). It is by far the most common type in the body. It has its own separate genetic code (different from that of the mother's). The critical thing to understand about chondral bone is that it's quite stubborn concerning the amount of growth it will express. Except for certain chemical exceptions such as growth hormones, vitamin D deficiencies, and rare defects, its development is strictly determined by the patient's personal genetic code. For example: You can drink all the milk in the world while growing up, but, unless you're genetically programmed to do so, you still won't end up seven feet tall. Sorry to break the news, but you'll never make the NBA on calcium intake alone.

There is a second type of bone in the body—known as *dermal bone*—that is different from the chondral variety in a very important way, especially as far as we dentists are concerned. Dermal bone looks like chondral bone. It's almost as hard as chondral bone. It feels, weighs, and even reproduces during healing like chondral bone. But there is one key difference: It doesn't always behave like chondral bone.

Dermal bone *isn't* stubborn; it *doesn't* always need to have its way. Put more scientifically, its growth is not strictly related to genetic determination. It is a "softer," more pliable type of bone, one that's developmentally more cooperative, forgiving, and even shapeable to a certain extent. With only a few exceptions, all of the bones of the face and the skull are made up of this type of bone, including the entire upper jaw (called the *maxilla*). Dermal bone is perfect for the skull since, as it grows, it will gently shape itself in order to conform and fit around finicky organs like the brain, the eyes, the internal ear, and the delicate balance structures of the inner ear.

Such highly specialized soft-tissue organs require precise specifications concerning their spacing in order to function properly. They need powerful protection, but they also need a certain amount of bony "breathing room." In other words, they can't tolerate physical pressure of any kind. Therefore, the protective bone enveloping them must develop in such a way as to adapt and fit, just right, to their particular anatomical shape (i.e., if the breathing room they need isn't exactly correct, there will be trouble).

Now, all of this isn't to say that dermal bone is soft and rubbery;

it's just about as hard as other types of bone. By saying it is "shapeable," I mean that it is pliable by certain types of unusual forces of a steady and persistent *hydraulic* or *mechanical* nature (i.e., forces that are capable of pushing gently on it over a long period of time, such as months or years). This is why children who suffer from a condition called *hydrocephaly* (too much fluid around the brain) develop such unusually large heads. In this condition, the patient's *cerebrospinal fluid*, which surrounds the outside of the brain and some of its inner portions, cannot properly drain from inside the skull. As this fluid slowly—but steadily—builds up, the *calvarium* (the upper part of the bony skull cap covering the brain) grows larger and larger in response to the abnormal pressure built up inside it. This is an example of how dermal bone, specialized for the head, can be improperly shaped by unusual forces of a hydraulic nature. Thus, dermal bone is very adaptable.

The adaptability and shape-conforming aspects of dermal bone can also be seen in its response to forces of a mechanical nature. A great illustration comes from the historical use of artificial *prostheses* (man-made body parts fabricated to replace missing arms, legs, eyes, and even teeth). A little-known example of this is the Venetian glass blowers of the Italian Renaissance.

Even though they had no comprehension of the biological principles behind it, these artisans were aware of the adaptability of dermal bone in the human face and knew how to take advantage of it. As experts of fabricating objects out of glass, they found that if a small child lost an eye—due to a traumatic accident or some other reason—they could create a convincing replica of the missing organ and insert it into the vacant eye socket. This, of course, would greatly improve the child's facial appearance. But as the child grew, something odd would occur: The natural, undamaged eye and its bony eye socket would grow increasingly larger, but the socket with the artificial eye would not. Consequently, the child would develop a distorted face with one eye socket smaller than the other, giving him or her a lopsided appearance. Even more interesting was the fact that, if every year or so they fashioned a progressively larger artificial replacement, they could gradually, and gently, force the vacated eye socket to grow on a pace similar to that of the natural eye and its own bony socket.

The result was an upper face that remained symmetrical. This phenomenon was only possible because of the adaptability of dermal bone. It wouldn't work on arms or legs, for example. (The only way an arm or leg can be artificially lengthened is through modern orthopedic surgical techniques. Human limbs are made up of chondral bone and, as such, lack the ability to conform and adapt to hydraulic or mechanical forces on their own.)

Perhaps all of this has started to seem a little boring right about now, but hang on! There is one last type of bone we should discuss, and it is—as far as orthodontics is concerned—the most important of them all.

This third type of bone is so peculiar that it doesn't even have a name of its own (science can be cruel!). In actuality, this third type is a hybrid of the first two—not a mixture, but rather a sandwich-like formation of chondral and dermal bone, each layer separate and distinct, one sitting atop the other. There are only two known examples in the entire body. The first is the *clavicle*, or collarbone—though nobody knows for sure why it's made of this type of bone. The second example is the one we're most interested in: the lower jaw.

The lower jaw is called the *mandible*. It is a horseshoe-shaped bone with bony hinges on each end called *condyles*. These rounded balls fit into sockets at the base of the skull back by the ears. The bulk of the mandible—including your chin, the lower base that slants toward your ears, the back lower corner by your neck, the broad section that rises to the base of your jaw socket, and almost all of the rounded condyles that hinge with your skull—is chondral in origin (as a reminder, chondral is the stubborn, genetically determined type, resistant to most outside influences). But the tooth-holding socket bone of the mandible—i.e., the bony socket that holds the roots of the lower teeth—is dermal, or shapeable, bone. This is a big deal. We'll see why shortly.

All of this comes together when you examine the causes of a malocclusion, or a bad bite, in which the teeth and jaws don't fit together properly. Jawbone shape and alignment play a very important role in various types of malocclusions (bad bites). It's not just the teeth and how they look that count anymore; how the bones are shaped and how the upper and lower jaws fit together, especially at full bite, turn out to be very important. Sometimes even serious, long-term health issues are at stake when the fit of the upper and lower teeth is improper—which, consequently, forces the jaw sockets to not work correctly. The result can be lasting jaw and facial pains as well as—and here's the big one—constantly recurring headaches!

TWO

How Braces Work: The Steel Feel

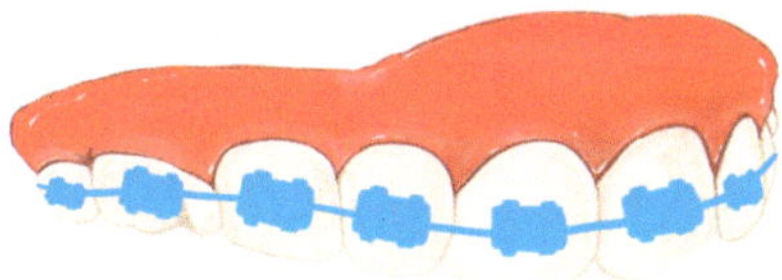

For what man would like to be true,
that he more readily believes.

— Sir Francis Bacon (1561–1626),
English lawyer, philosopher, and essayist

In the dental vernacular, metal braces are referred to as *fixed appliances.*

Now, when we say the word appliance, we don't mean a stove or a refrigerator; rather, we're alluding to any device, retainer, brace, wire, etc., that is placed on or around the teeth with some sort of orthodontic purpose. It "applies" energy to the system (in this case, the mouth). Similarly, if you say the word *fixed* to an auto mechanic, it means the car will start; to a boxing promoter, it means the outcome of a fight is known ahead of time; to a politician, that the election is rigged. But to a dentist, the word fixed means anything that is glued onto the teeth and is designed to be removable only by the dentist. Hence the terms *fixed crowns* (caps), *fixed bridgework*, and *fixed appliances*.

Orthodontic appliances such as retainers, splints, etc., are not fixed but are instead removable and can easily be put in or taken out by either the patient or the dentist. But more on those later.

Fixed appliances—or metal braces—have been the mainstay of traditional American orthodontics for more than a hundred years. There are all sorts of subtypes, but, for right now, that isn't important. What *is* important is that these types of appliances—for the most part—essentially move teeth *through* the stationary socket bone (called the *alveolar processes*) of the upper or lower jaws. This happens because the braces, activated by a wire, spring, or rubber elastic of some sort, impart mechanical energy to the tooth or teeth in question by means of a little clip called a *bracket*. Each bracket is a small metal fitting attached directly to the tooth, usually by a special whiz-bang dental adhesive. The mechanical force imparted by the combination of wire, spring, elastic, and metal bracket travels through the crown of the tooth—to which orthodontic brackets are directly attached—then down the hard root into the bony socket. As a result, the bone of the socket wall will be pressured by that side of the root, which causes part of the socket bone to slowly dissolve. This allows the tooth in question to be shifted slightly into a new location, made possible by the dissolved bone adjacent to the tooth root. Simultaneously, new bone then grows in the space created by this shift in position, filling in the opposite side of the tooth root.

So, there you have it. You can start with a tooth in position A (over here) and can move it to position B (over there) by the application of a steady mechanical force from an orthodontic brace, which will gradually dissolve the bone around the roots and move those roots—and, thus, the entire tooth itself—slowly but surely right through the stationary bone of the jaw.

The big thing to understand here is that traditional metal braces, for the most part, move teeth through stationary jaw bone without doing much to change the shape of the jaw itself or—much more importantly—the front-to-back bony alignment of the stationary upper jaw to the highly movable lower jaw. Additionally, fixed appliances don't do anything to change the size or length of the muscles of the jaws (which is sometimes important, other times not). However, we now know that the jaw muscles sometimes *do* require changing. Which means metal braces aren't always enough, and other types of appliances are needed. And now we have them! Even more exciting is that these orthodontic devices for changing "crooked" muscles are *not* fixed—they're removable!

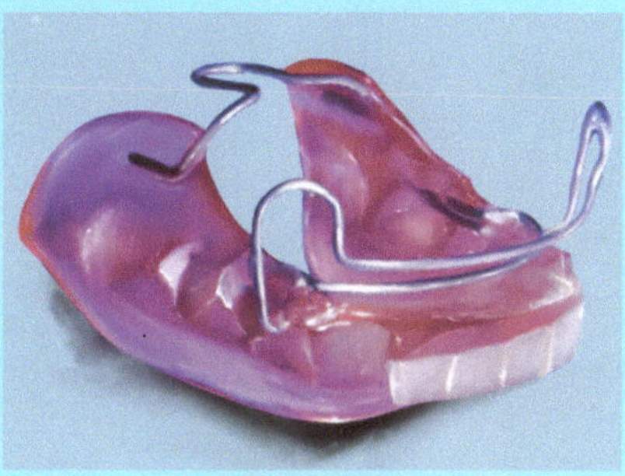

Figure 2 - 1 (A)

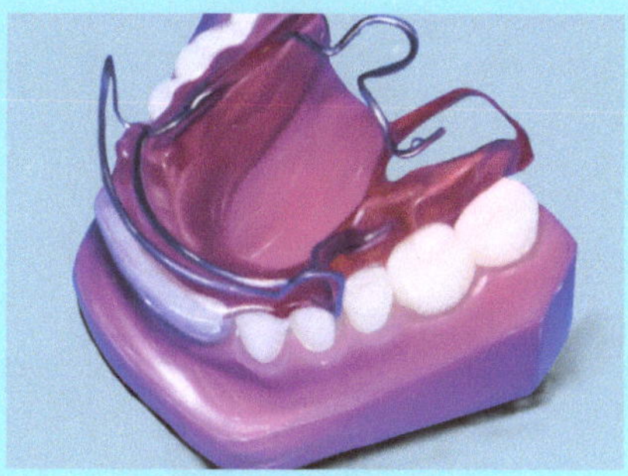

Figure 2 - 1 (B)

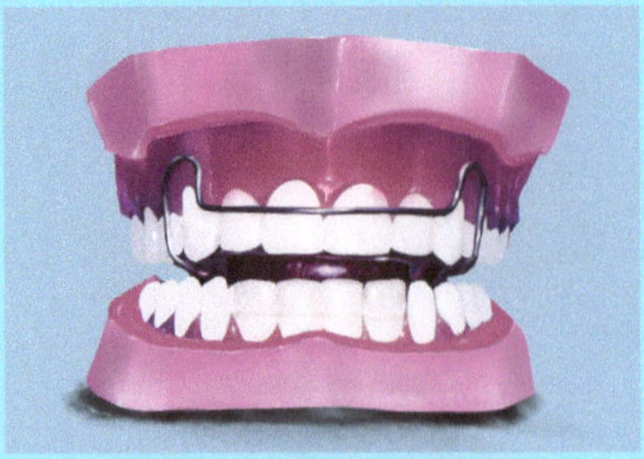

Figure 2 - 2 (A)

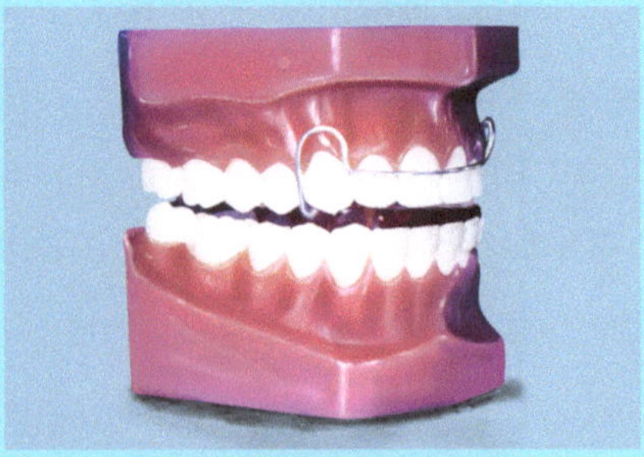

Figure 2 - 2 (B)

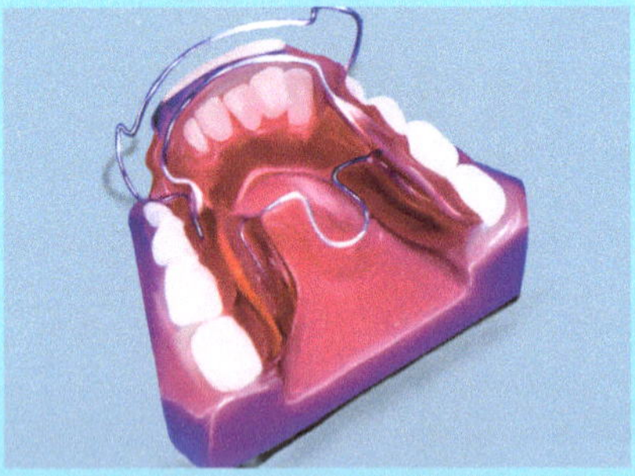

Figure 2 - 3 (A)

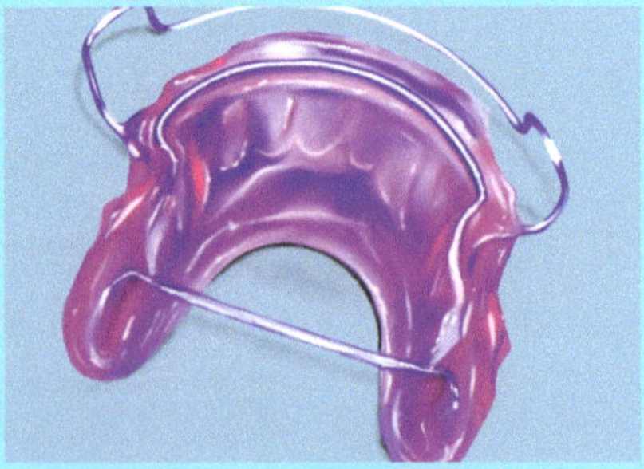

Figure 2 - 3 (B)

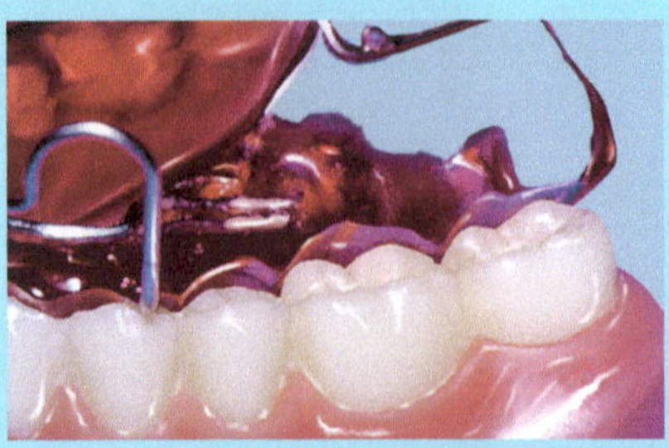

Figure 2 - 4 (A)

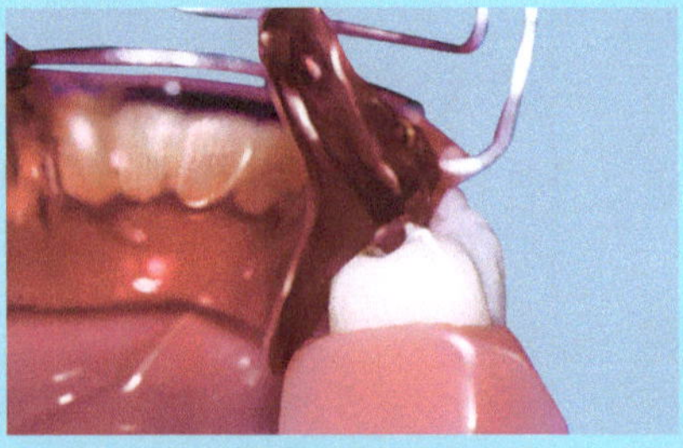

Figure 2 - 4 (B)

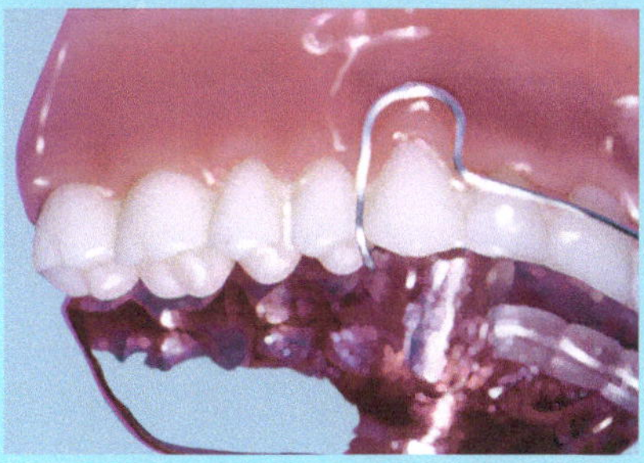

Figure 2 - 5 (A)

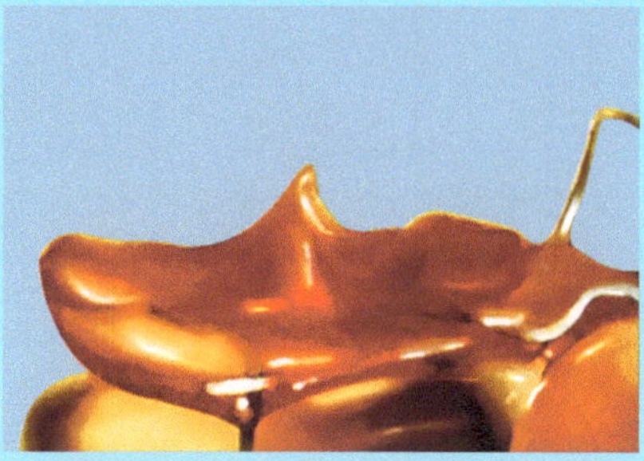

Figure 2 - 5 (B)

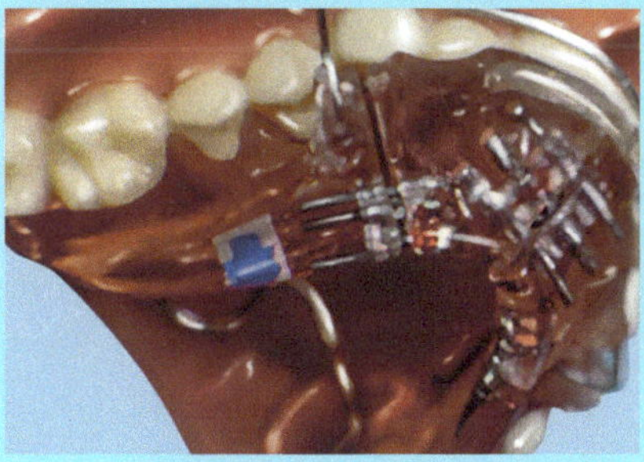

Figure 2 - 6 (A)

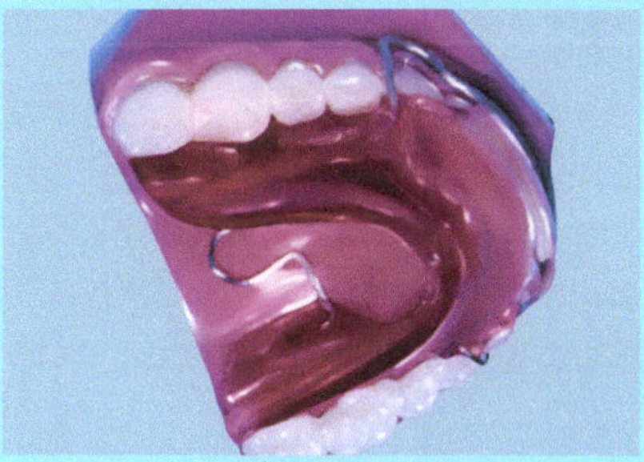

Figure 2 - 6 (B)

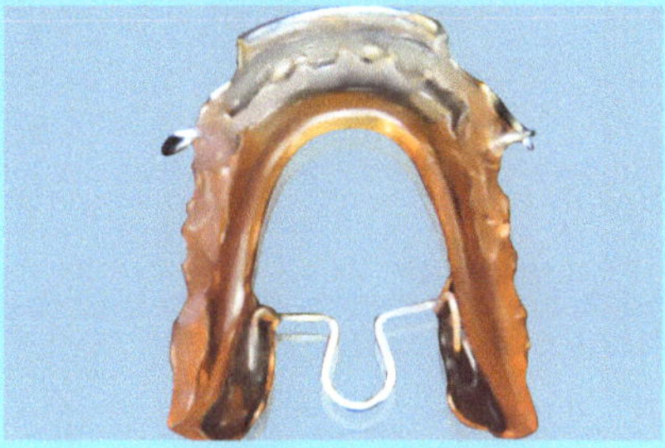

Figure 2 - 7 (A)

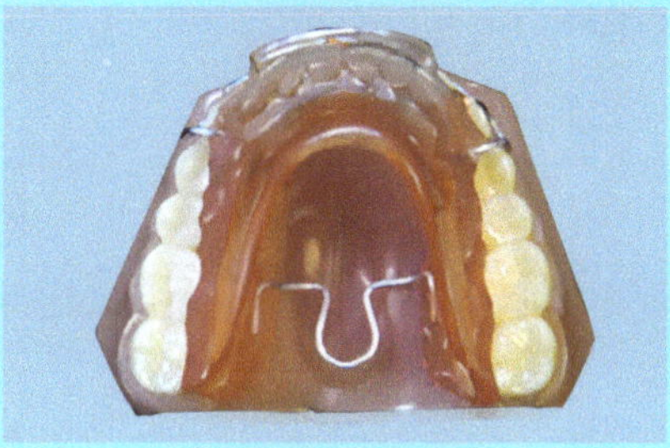

Figure 2 - 7 (B)

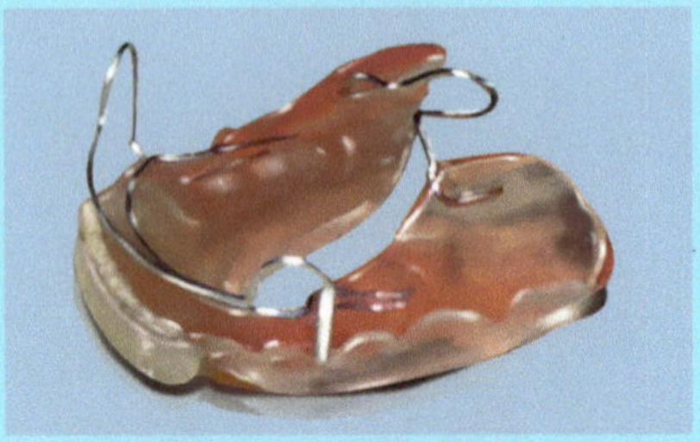

Figure 2 - 8 (A)

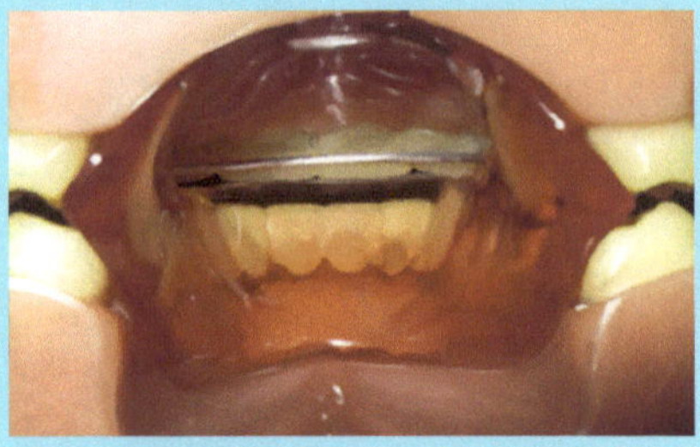

Figure 2 - 8 (B)

→ Everybody knows what fixed (or glued on) metal braces look like; no pictures are needed for that. But do you know what removable functional appliances look like? Here are some images, which depict inside-out, up-and-down, and front-and-back views of one of the most famous functional appliances of all time. It's called a Bionator, and was perfected by a German orthodontist by the name of Wilhelm Balters during the 1960s. Although he modified and refined what were, at the time, more primitive versions, the Bionator's origins date back to appliances invented in Norway over 50 years earlier. They were okay, though not nearly as effective as later iterations. But, they were a starting point, and doctors from all over Europe proceeded to work on many different designs, some of which were pretty crude. When the Bionator finally arrived on the scene, it was initially referred to as the "miracle appliance," because it did what was believed, at the time, to be impossible. Nobody really knew for sure how to move a backward-sitting lower jaw forward (i.e., nobody knew how to "grow chins," or correct the improperly working jaw muscles that held such a jaw too far back). Functional appliances, worn only 16-20 hours per day, can do this!

Note: Some of these photos include Bionators with expansion screws in their bottom portions, which are sometimes used for technical reasons.

So, for example, if your child's particular type of malocclusion is one that exhibits straight, properly shaped bones and "straight," properly sized jaw muscles but exhibits misaligned or crooked teeth, then traditional metal braces will work great! That's all you'll need to correctly treat the case. But if the upper or lower jawbones themselves are crooked, misshapen, or, most importantly, misaligned front to back, upper jaw to lower jaw, or if the jaw musculature that surrounds and operates the bones is either improperly functioning (twisted, if you will) or *foreshortened* (being shorter than they actually should be), then a metal brace treatment is often seriously handicapped as to what it can accomplish.

Metal braces—nearly the only thing used in American-style orthodontics for the past hundred years—can't change the jaw muscles, and neither can they easily, if ever, change the jawbones' front-to-back, top-to-bottom, functional alignment. (This has a lot to do with ultimate facial appearance and the beauty of the smile line once the metal braces come off). Yet many children have serious problems with both areas. So if you're a dental professional doing braces, and you are forced to deal with crooked teeth accompanied by misaligned jawbones and "crooked" jaw muscles, how do you handle such problems, when the only thing at your disposal is a treatment technique that can't quite do the job? The only alternative left open to you isn't a pleasant one: You're forced to fudge. Let's examine how some treating clinicians used to do it.

THREE

The Great "In-Your-Face" Extraction Fight

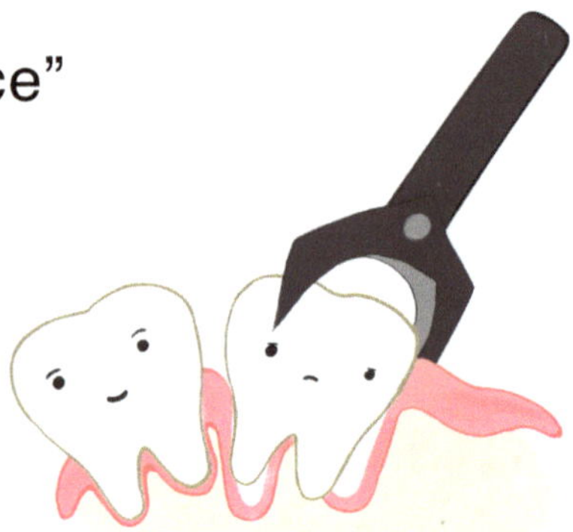

Is it progress when a cannibal uses a knife and a fork?

— Stanislaw Jerzy Lec (1909–1966), Polish poet

Dentists clump crooked bites, or malocclusions, into three broad categories: Class I, Class II, and Class III (dentists aren't always very colorful in their namings). These three groupings are classified according to how the teeth and jaws align.

A *Class I malocclusion* refers to the type of bite where the upper and lower jaws—as well as the teeth—line up pretty good on a horizontal basis when the patient's face is viewed in profile and he or she is fully biting down (complete habitual biting on all back teeth). In a Class I-type malocclusion, only the teeth themselves are a little twisted or overlapped in their respective sockets.

Alternatively, a *Class II malocclusion*—by far the most common—is one in which almost all the lower teeth (*Dental Class II*), and even the entire lower jaw itself (*Skeletal Class II*), will align too far behind the upper teeth and upper jaw at full closure. Both types of Class II bites (dental and skeletal) can result in a horizontal misalignment between the upper and lower front teeth, which can be quite unsightly. It makes the upper front teeth appear (notice I use the word *appear*) overly protruded, resulting in the common nickname "buck teeth." Surprisingly, this condition is almost invariably due to insufficient forward growth in the mandible. Jaw muscles that don't work quite right can cause the lower jaw to not grow large enough or forward enough. Hence the child's lower jaw bites too far back, and his or her chin area looks retruded and weak.

The third category, the *Class III malocclusion*, is relatively rare and exhibits a lower jaw that is usually too protruded to fit properly with its counterpart (imagine Jay Leno). These skeletal malocclusions are due to excessive lower jawbone growth that makes it too long relative to the upper jaw.

It is the Class II malocclusion that lies at the heart of all recent orthodontic advancements in treatment. The old ways of fixing it weren't so hot; the new ways, however, have produced spectacular results (which we'll look at here soon enough).

For the formidable skeletal-type (more severe) Class II malocclusion, there can be no doubt as to what's happening. The entire lower jaw—teeth and all—aligns and bites too far back, making it underdeveloped, diminished, weak-looking, and just plain unattractive in general facial appearance, especially in profile. Again, as malocclusions go, this is a common problem, yet certain types of it have fooled orthodontic specialists for generations.

To the early, traditional orthodontic world, a sizable Class II malocclusion of the skeletal variety was a devil. It caused all sorts of treatment difficulties, and nobody really knew what to do with it. They could move the teeth with metal braces, but, no matter how hard they tried, they just couldn't seem to get that retruded, underdeveloped, backward-biting lower jaw to grow out more forward. Consequently, they concluded it couldn't be done. Some believed that removing certain permanent teeth might help solve the problem—as well as other orthodontic issues, the biggest of which was excessive "jumbling" or overcrowding of teeth within jaws that were seemingly too small.

And that's where the "fudge factor" came in.

The teeth slated for extraction were almost invariably either the first or second permanent bicuspids. As you'll remember, these beautiful, graceful teeth reside on the sides of the dental arches between the six front incisors (called *centrals*, *laterals*, and cuspids—or "eye teeth," for extra credit) and the big, heavy-duty grinding molars in the back. The bicuspids occupy a spot on the dental arch equivalent to the corners of the mouth on the smile line. This simple fact is what forms the basis for one of the most important and valid criticisms of the *bicuspid extraction* orthodontic technique, which was (and sometimes still is) used to gain empty space in the dental arches to help unjumble and more easily realign the remaining teeth. This technique can produce adverse effects on the face and the beauty of the smile: It can result in too much empty space at the extraction site, and, hence, over-shrinkage of the finished dental arches.

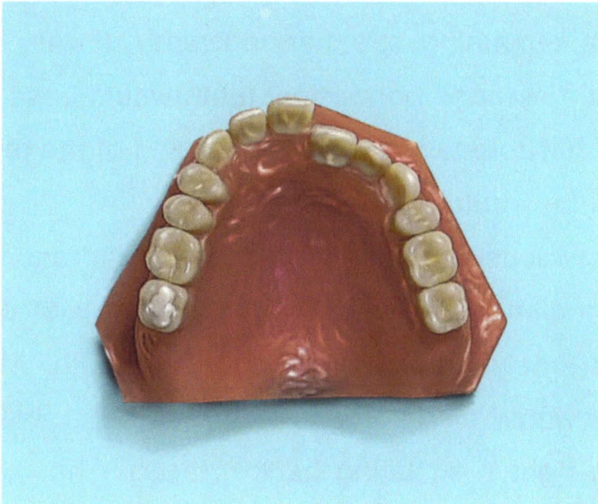

3-1

→ Figure 3-1: This plastic model of an upper jaw with its dental arch of teeth is a side-by-side comparison of the difference in arch length, front to back, between an arch with both bicuspids present vs. an arch of the same-sized teeth with only one bicuspid present. At the world meeting of the European Orthodontic Society in Florence, Italy, a number of years back, research was presented that showed that, in finished cases involving the extraction of bicuspids, upper front teeth were positioned, on average, 7 millimeters further back. Lower front teeth, meanwhile, were positioned an average of 3.5 millimeters back, in relation to their normal bite. Imagine what that might do to the fullness and beauty of a patient's smile—not to mention what it might do to the anatomical support for those lips, which are then draped over the over-retracted post-treatment front teeth, thus affecting the entire facial profile and smile line.

Note: The average width of a bicuspid is about 7 millimeters.

When first proposed almost a hundred years ago, the use of the bicuspid extraction technique was embraced by many early orthodontists with open arms. It made correcting horrific malocclusions much easier and faster than the alternative of trying to force those crooked teeth to fit into undersized or deformed jaws. Removal of the bicuspids also helped with the post-treatment stability of the remaining straightened teeth. It was believed that extracting some of these permanent teeth would ease the pressure and strain so that *relapse* (a slow rebounding of the teeth back to a crooked position) would be much less likely.

Extracting bicuspids, one from each quadrant, seemed like the perfectly logical thing to do when dealing with dental arches that were extremely crowded with jumbled teeth. Many felt that this technique would also somehow correct the problem of a lower jaw not biting right (i.e., biting back too far). Thus the pendulum of orthodontic opinion took its first big swing, favoring the bicuspid extraction technique. For a long while, it even looked as if it was good enough to stick around. But guess what: As the bicuspid extraction technique came under repeated scrutiny—and after additional study of a vast number of cases that had been treated with the technique—it became clear to many dentists that this approach might not represent the "end-all, be-all" it was originally cracked up to be. There were too many problems—serious ones!

One of the major issues was that, once the treatment was completed and the metal braces came off, with four permanent bicuspid teeth now missing, the patient was sometimes left with a "sunken-in" appearance to his or her face. This was due to a lack of foundational lip support as well as a lack of the lips' usual plumpness. Although the remaining teeth were aligned and looked straight, each upper and lower dental arch was now smaller in size by two teeth, one premolar on the right and one premolar on the left for both the upper and lower dental arches. This reduction caused a dramatic loss in lip support, as the corners of the mouth were usually supported by these now-missing bicuspids. The paradox involved with the bicuspid extraction technique was that the more protruded the upper teeth were in the beginning—and the more jumbled they were before the braces were applied—the better the method seemed to work. Conversely, in certain cases, the less serious malocclusions were the ones with resulting disfigurements to the lips, smile line, and face. And therein lay a dilemma for early orthodontists.

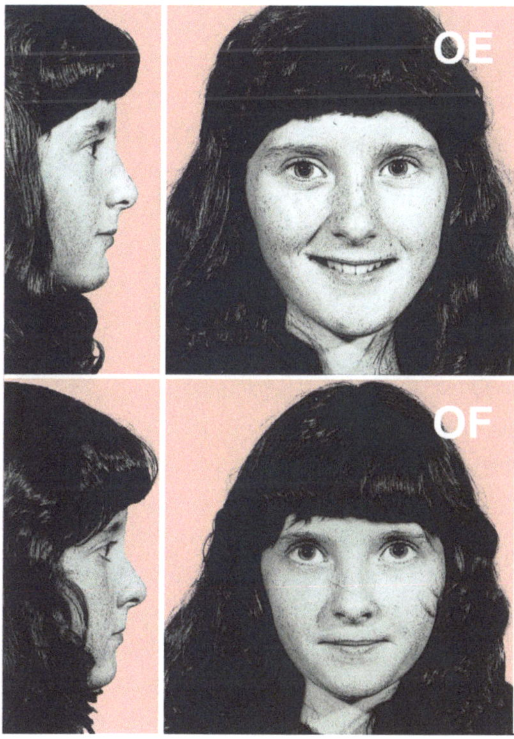

(A)

→ Figure 3-2 (A): Here are some pictures of a pair of identical twins who were treated orthodontically by my friend and colleague Dr. Hans Eirew, a British orthodontist who practiced in Manchester, England. Nicknamed "the Eirew twins," they both possessed identical malocclusions.

Since this case took place many years ago, back when second-molar extraction techniques were just appearing on the scene, the decision was made to treat one of the twins using the usual traditional bicuspid extraction technique, while the other was treated using newer functional orthodontic and orthopedic methods—all in an attempt to see how each would affect the final outcome. The twin in the image marked OE received the traditional metal braces/bicuspid extraction treatment. The twin in the image labeled OF received the functional appliance-type treatment (with just a brief period of metal braces, in order to "touch up" the final tooth angulation). Remember, these pictures are of two different people.

However, in the intervening months of orthodontic treatment, something happened. The first twin (OE) noticed she'd gradually begun looking less and less like her sister, who was receiving the alternative functional appliance treatment. In fact, OE became so distraught over the disparity in appearance that Dr. Eirew had to stop treatment before the case was even finished. (That's why, if you look closely, you'll notice some of her remaining teeth still seem a little twisted and aren't perfectly straight.)

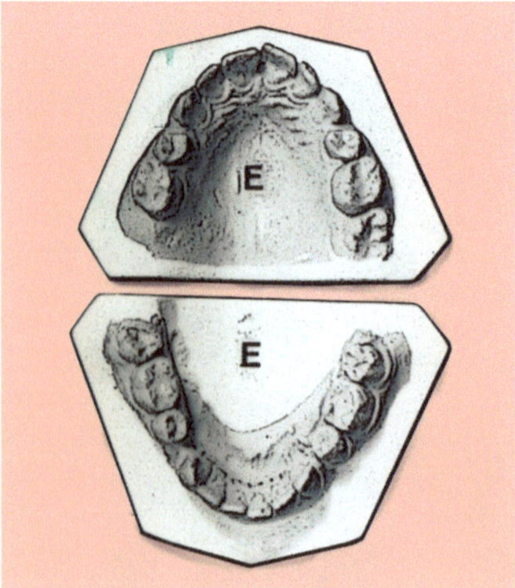

(B)

→ Figure 3-2 (B): Final appearance of the size and shape of the upper and lower dental arches of OE, who received the metal brace/bicuspid extraction-type treatment.

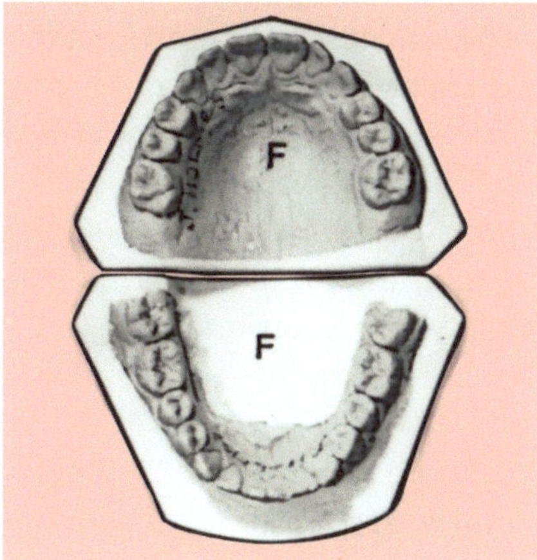

(C)

→ Figure 3-2 (C): The final appearance of the upper and lower dental arches of OF, who received the functional appliance-type treatment.

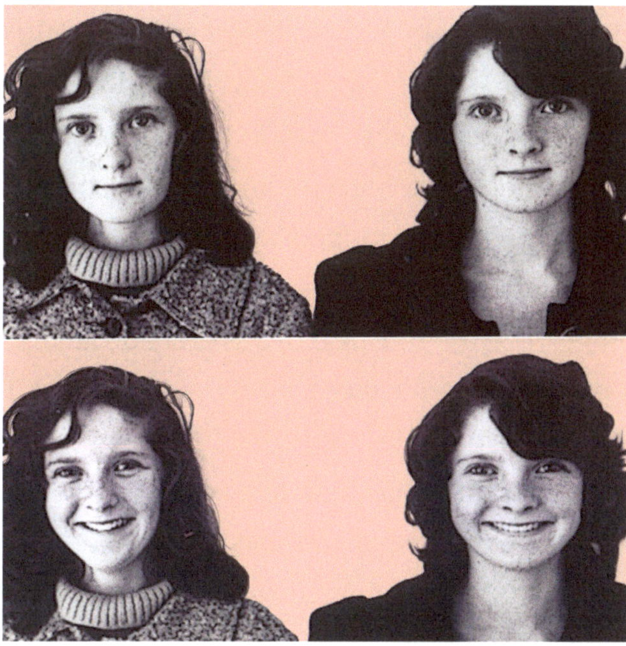

(D)

→ Figure 3-2 (D): Final comparison of the post-treatment results between the identical twins (extraction vs. non-extraction).

Note: When these photographs appeared in my first textbook, *The Clinical Management of Basic Maxillofacial Orthopedic Appliances, Volume I: Mechanics* (1986), hostile critics remarked that the only thing these pictures proved was that "our British colleagues" did not do a very good job on the twin who received traditional metal braces and extraction. (Remember: OE wanted treatment stopped *before* Dr. Eirew could finish the case. Oh, and by the way, Dr. Eirew was, at one time, the president of the prestigious British Orthodontic Society—i.e., no slouch!

For a case of limited dental crowding exhibiting a Class I jaw-to-jaw relationship—i.e., a mild malocclusion with nicely shaped and aligned jawbones, properly functioning jaw muscles, and only a few twisted or crooked teeth—obviously there existed no need to extract any teeth at all. The non-extraction method of doing the braces worked out fine. Put the braces on. Straighten the teeth. That was it.

And for a case—again, with Class I jaws—where the upper and lower teeth had become crowded too far forward, with the incisors protruding out (true buck teeth) and with both the upper and lower bicuspids and molars drifted way forward from their normal positions and piling up in the front like a chain-reaction car wreck on a California freeway, the bicuspid extraction technique did, at times, work out fine. (Here's more extra credit for you: These kinds of malocclusions, where the teeth are both jumbled up *and* truly stick out way too far, are known as *bimaxillary protrusions.* In order to better justify the extraction of four bicuspids, a lot of orthodontists call a particular malocclusion they're treating a bimaxillary protrusion. However, true crooked teeth of this type are quite rare.)

The trouble started when orthodontists were faced with how best to handle the "in-between" types of malocclusions (i.e., the ones that only exhibit a moderate degree of jumbled teeth and maybe only a slight Class II skeletal configuration). The problem was a dental dilemma. Should the poor orthodontist try to shoehorn all those teeth into slightly undersized and misaligned jaws, thus risking strain on those tightly fitted teeth? Such strain, after all, could leave those teeth vulnerable to severe relapse and to the eventual collapse of the straightened dental arches. Or, should that orthodontist take out four bicuspids—one in each quadrant at the corners of the smile line—thereby creating excess space? What if only a little extra space was needed? Too bad: You can't take out half or a fourth of a tooth; it's all or none!

Furthermore, would shrinking that extra extraction-site free space with additional brace work end up over-retracting the front teeth and "caving-in" the proper lip support they'd have normally provided, thereby ruining the beauty and fullness of the lips/smile?

Tough decisions, indeed.

Another hitch that was added to all this was what to do when—on top of having crooked, jumbled, and crowded teeth—the patient also exhibited a severe Skeletal Class II retruded lower jaw with a resultant seven-, eight-, or ten-millimeter horizontal gap between the (seemingly) protruded upper front teeth and the recessed lower front incisors (or an entire recessed lower jaw).

Not only did they have to extract as many as four bicuspids to get the teeth constricted together (again, accomplished through subsequent brace work), but they also had to force the upper front teeth far enough back to pair, during biting, with the lower front incisors. Those incisors, in turn, could be even more retruded because they were sitting in a mandible that was itself positioned too far back in a "galloping" Class II state of underdevelopment. In our business, that's a really big gap to try to close up.

Moreover, extracting bicuspids and using metal braces to treat these types of cases the "traditional way" often resulted in a very collapsed, sunken smile, one characterized by a weak-looking retruded chin and a "dished-in" facial profile. Folks, we have to be honest with ourselves here: In extreme cases, as far as facial appearances go, those types of smiles are simply less attractive than a fully filled-out "normal" smile.

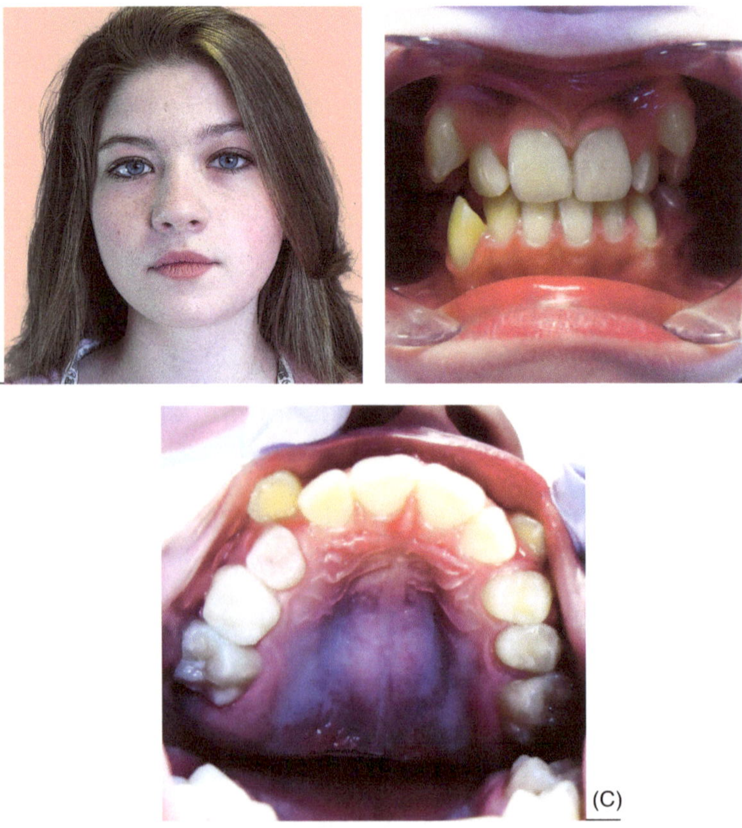

(A) (B) (C)

→ Figures 3-3 (A - C): These pre-treatment photos show a teenage girl with four totally "blocked out" upper and lower, right and left, adult cuspids. The traditional metal braces-type treatment usually included the extraction of four bicuspids to make room for those cuspids in their proper place along the dental arch—which would then only be followed, years later, by the additional surgical extraction of all four wisdom teeth when the patient was in his or her late teens or early twenties (in other words: eight adult teeth relegated to the disposal bin). Thanks to modern second molar-extraction principles, only four teeth need to be extracted, and the finished orthodontic result almost invariably provides superior facial aesthetic results.

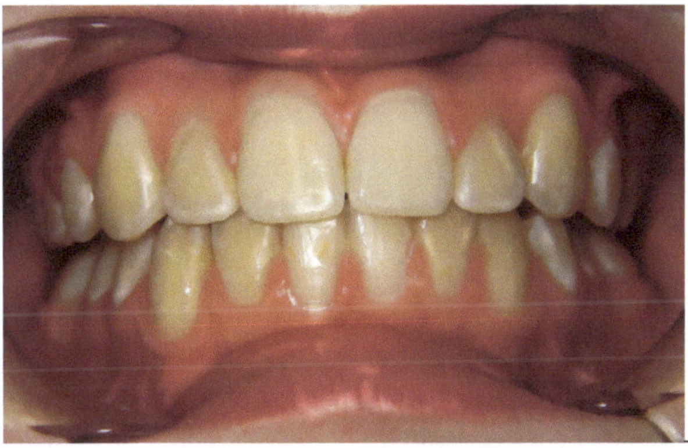

(D)

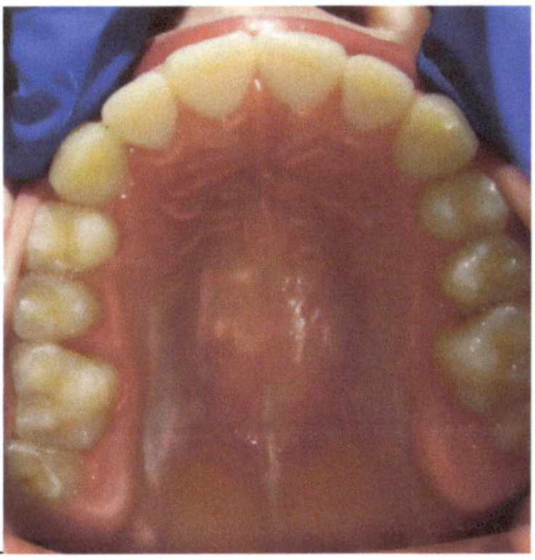

(E)

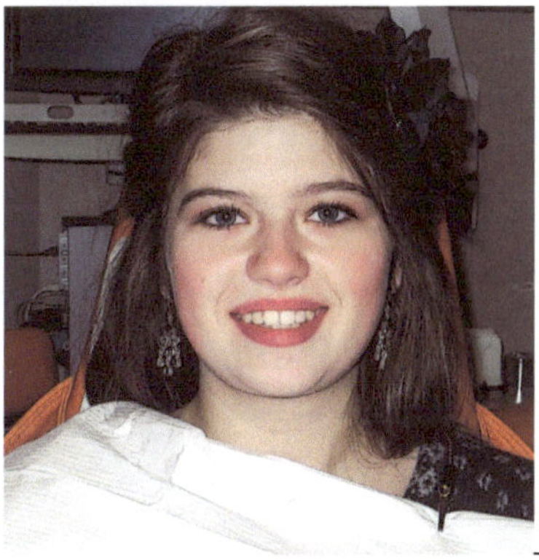

(F)

→ Figures 3-3 (D - F): Observe the beautiful post-treatment results thanks to the second molar-extraction techniques! There are very complicated technical reasons why these methods are, in many ways, better for the jaw joints. (Notice how, in Figure 3-3 [E], all four premolars are present and assisting with proper lip support and the fullness of the smile. The four wisdom teeth will erupt in the months to come and will occupy the spaces left over from the extracted second molars. Cool, huh?)

This is why orthodontists have developed numerous tooth-moving orthodontic techniques over the years in an effort to shrink the bicuspid extraction-site space with minimum retraction of the front teeth, lips, smile line, and lower facial profile. Sometimes these deleterious side effects to the face were adequately concealed; for those patients, things often turned out reasonably well. Sometimes, however, those side effects *weren't* sufficiently hidden, and patients dealt with the consequences for life. That's why, in the years since, orthodontic clinicians have developed all sorts of clever little tricks to use in conjunction with metal braces and (hopefully) avoid this problem.

Be that as it may, orthodontists back then regularly used the bicuspid extraction technique on severe Skeletal Class II cases (where the lower jaw is too short and too far back) because the limitations inherent in metal braces forced them to do the best they could with what little they had. Unfortunately, for some cases, this turned out to be the wrong tool for the job. The metal wires and braces, as good as they were at moving teeth, were basically an *orthodontic* technique (tooth alignment) trying to solve what was actually an *orthopedic* (bone alignment) and *myofunctional* (muscle alignment) problem.

So, while they made the teeth appear straight, the upper and lower jaws and their passenger dental arches were not always aligned when the patient closed their teeth in full bite. The distorted jaw muscles (which couldn't be seen) were not always corrected back to normal either. The poor orthodontists who only had metal braces to work with were often forced to fit the teeth to the deformed and/or misaligned top-to-bottom set of jaws. And if the jaws were misaligned at the bone- and muscle-level from the outset, then they were often still crooked when the metal brace-type orthodontic treatment was completed, regardless of how straight and dentally aligned the teeth looked on the surface.

Those early dentists and orthodontists did their best. It was a noble effort. They disguised the issues pretty well by lining up the teeth so that they appeared straight (in both the bite and the fit), but the upper and lower jawbones (in which the teeth were lodged) were still misaligned in many cases. So, in the final analysis, those clinicians just plain fudged.

But the worst outcome by far had nothing to do with looks. It had to do with pain—terrible pain. In those kinds of situations, where the lower jaw is forced to bite back too far and doesn't line up properly with the upper jaw during biting and chewing, there are often resultant side effects: *chronic* (long-term), *recurrent* (frequent), tension-type headaches, and/or migraines as well as a facial-pain condition known by the slang term *TMD*. But, for now, we're only discussing how things used to be done, back when nobody in the lay community—nor even a major part of the dental population—was aware of the orthodontic-TMD relationship. Back then, the term TMD meant a little something different to dentists, and thus they viewed it on a much smaller screen.

New knowledge and techniques, however, now allow us to properly correct these hidden upper-to-lower jawbone and jaw muscle problems, which have, in a sneaky type of orthopedic bony disguise, plagued orthodontic treatment from the very beginning. This new, more advanced knowledge is good for everybody. It's not a matter of emotion. It's not a matter of choice. It is just cold, hard science!

FOUR

Fun with Functional Appliances: The Plastic Fantastic

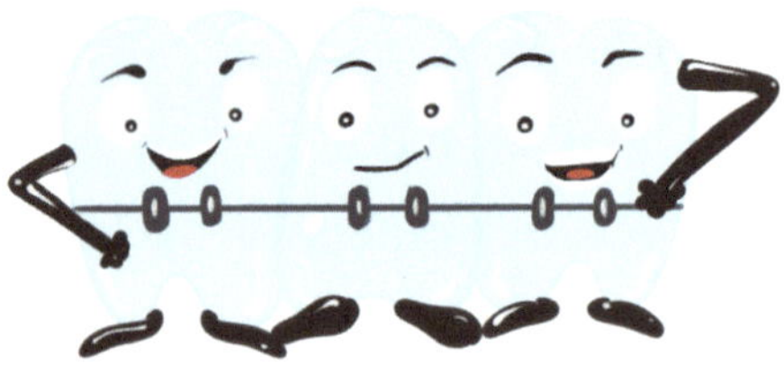

That is the essence of science: ask an impertinent question, and you are on your way to a pertinent answer.

— Jacob Bronowski (1908–1974),
Polish-born mathematician and humanist

By now, the number of difficulties orthodontists have faced (no pun intended) in dealing with the staggering problems of treating malocclusions—which can feature various combinations of crooked teeth and misaligned jaws—should be clear. All in all, those professionals have done a fine job. But there *are* problems.

Essentially, all they had to work with were metal braces, which only moved teeth through otherwise stationary upper and lower jawbones. They couldn't move the lower jaw itself from a retruded, skeletal, backward-biting Class II relationship to a more proper, straight, up-and-down Class I relationship. If it was askew before orthodontic treatment began, the bony jaw-to-jaw alignment—front-to-back, functional lower jaw to upper jaw—had to be disguised by the mere movement of the teeth alone.

Nor could early orthodontists deal with certain aspects of the "crooked" musculature of the jaws that surrounded and operated it all. Many of them never truly understood the real significance (and power) of that surrounding musculature. Remember, the vast majority of malocclusions result not only from teeth that can't seem to line themselves up correctly, but also from an improper jaw muscle environment that can warp the shape of the jawbones and even distort and misalign the whole jaw system. (Why, exactly, the muscles do this is an entirely separate story. Don't ask; it's too complicated to get into right now. It's enough to know that, sometimes, they just do.)

Early orthodontists often were forced to try to make the teeth fit each other and somehow stay straight while sitting in what were, at their foundations, essentially crooked jaws. Sometimes this forced dental clinicians to extract perfectly good teeth at the corners of the mouth. Many times, this led to a detrimental effect on the face's final appearance as well as on the fullness and beauty of the smile, leaving it lacking in normal lip support and plumpness.

When the braces were removed, the "orthodontic look"—as it's sometimes called—robbed many a young man of that strong, handsome appearance, and it denied many a beautiful young lady that opulent and attractive "pouty" lip line for which movie stars, supermodels, and beauty contest winners are so famous. Through it all, many clinicians felt there had to be a better way than just cranking on crooked teeth with steel wires and metal braces until those teeth could be forced out of their natural bony sockets to new places in the jaws. There had to be something better than the mere illusion of straightness and proper dental alignment.

Consider this: No animal known to man has ever had to have its teeth straightened or removed to allow the others to fit within its jaws correctly. Have you ever seen a cat or a dog—or a horse or a cow—with crooked teeth? Of course not. Man is the only animal that suffers from malocclusions. Why? A plethora of reasons exist, some of which are too complicated to go into here. For starters, we don't even know all the reasons. It's not just one thing that causes crooked teeth and/or anatomically distorted jaws, but rather several factors acting in concert to produce that final jumbled dental mess. Things like nutrition, pollution, breathing obstruction, swallowing problems, and premature loss of baby teeth are just a few of the contributors (as is genetics—although to a lesser degree than originally believed).

With only one kind of technique available to them, the American orthodontic community admirably struggled on through the early and middle 20th century encased in their own private and clinically exclusive scientific kingdom. They were flush with the thrill of the tooth-moving powers they felt they had at their disposal; in their own shortsighted view of things, they were adamant in saying their method of treatment was the best—if not the only—way to treat malocclusions in children. They were supremely confident they could straighten out just about any kind of crooked bite. All seemed well and in order. Theirs was a standard for the world! They were on fire with it. And, much of the time, they did a great job.

"But colder eyes quietly watched from a distance." The system had its critics, detractors whose shrewd dental perceptions recognized the inherent flaws in the American orthodontic approach.

Things in the world of braces were starting to "cook on the orthodontic backburners." New ideas were germinating—something better *could* be done for these types of cases. Help was on the way!

Enter the Europeans. Some of our colleagues across the pond had developed a different way of looking at the world of crooked teeth. Although it took them generations to evolve these alternative ideas, they eventually came up with a revolutionary way of attacking bite deformities and treating malocclusions. This new approach can best be symbolized by the concept of the *maxillofacial triangle*. Admittedly, it's an intimidating-sounding name, but it's actually a very easy concept to understand, especially by the average layperson. Metal braces now had a new friend!

One of the old Latin-rooted terms for a jaw is *maxilla* in the singular and *maxillae* in the plural, and the complete anatomy of the face and jaws is referred to as the *maxillofacial complex*. One of the great, practical dental ideas of modern times is that all malocclusions of crooked teeth and bad bites may be thought of as conceptual triangles of improperly arranged—and, as a result, improperly functioning—teeth, bone, and muscle. Hence, the analogy of a triangle. The Americans conquered the tooth part of the triangle, but some of the great early European orthodontic researchers and clinicians attacked the malocclusion triangle from the other two sides, directing their energies to correcting the bone/muscle aspects of the various types of malocclusions also.

The results of their collective theories and clinical observations were twofold. First, there was a big difference between an orthodontically twisted, misplaced, or crooked set of teeth versus a merely crowded or jumbled set. Plain-old crooked teeth—as in twisted, tilted, or otherwise physically displaced individual teeth—were easily treatable with standard American-style metal braces and wires. Crowded teeth, on the other hand, were something a bit different. They were the result of being jumbled up and "squished together," instead of appearing in a nicely aligned dental arch pattern. This phenomenon occurred because the jaws into which these teeth were supposed to erupt were themselves too small. Or, the jawbones also were individually warped or misaligned. Stationary top jaw to moveable bottom jaw alignment was too far off to properly hold the teeth in place during chewing.

To this, the Americans figuratively laughed and said, "We know this. That's why we take teeth (the bicuspids) out at the corners of the mouth to make enough room for the unpressured straightening of the rest." The Europeans responded with their second big conclusion. Figuratively, they said, "Now, wait a minute. The reason the jaws don't grow big enough or line up right, teeth-wise, in correctly chewing/biting fashion is because the jawbones themselves are gradually warped and distorted from their normal shape/alignment due to overpowering, misdirecting jaw muscles, which constantly act on those tender, pliable jawbones while the child is still growing."

This process would result in a minor—or sometimes major—distorted shape or misalignment of the jawbones themselves. The European dentists reasoned further that if you could somehow strategically redirect those restrictive jaw muscle forces and cause them to pull on those growing bones in a more favorable direction, then, over time, the jaws could be made to grow naturally, straight and full like they're supposed to. By doing so, those jaws would be of a sufficient size and proper upper-to-lower alignment so as to permit the unrestrained, normal eruption of the mouth's permanent adult teeth.

At first, only the scientific elite of Europe attempted to understand, design, and use these removable functional appliances, and even these pioneering experts had great difficulties with them. The earliest designs were just too slow and inefficient. But the European dentists were a clever and observant bunch. They persisted in perfecting the technique because they knew, collectively, that they were onto something. In America, however, these functional appliances suffered a less than glorious debut.

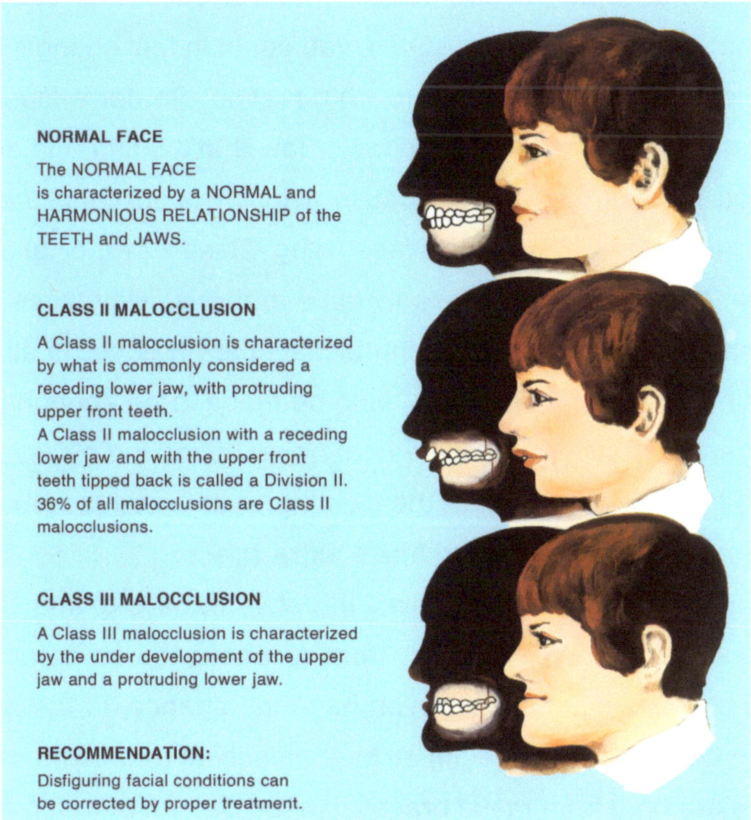

4-1

→ Figure 4-1: Drawings depicting the three major classifications of bites (occlusions) and the upper-jaw-to-lower-jaw relationships associated with them (Class I, Class II, Class III).

(Continued)

Notice how in the Class II bite all the lower teeth are further back behind the uppers (lower vertical red line behind the higher vertical red line). In the Class III bite, the lower teeth are too far in front of the upper teeth (the "Jay Leno look"). Class III types are not very common in the general population (about 6%). Major Class III bites are only treatable by means of *orthognathic* (jawbone) surgery.

Used correctly, functional appliances could remove the disfiguring Skeletal Class II mandibular retrusion of the lower jaw. By changing those jaw muscle forces that surround and continually "work on" those growing jawbones, you could in fact change the entire childhood lower jawbone growth direction. So, for a muscularly (and dentally) trapped, retruded lower jaw that's biting and aligning itself too far back, you could cause it to grow out more naturally forward into its normal, lower-face-filling Class I proper alignment position. You wouldn't necessarily have to throw away those gracefully shaped and smile-enhancing bicuspid teeth either to allow the remaining ones to fit. The jaws could be made large enough to hold the patient's existing teeth instead of doing things the old way—i.e., making the patient's teeth fit the existing undersized jaws by eliminating some of those teeth to make extra space.

With undersized lower jaws thereby made big and straight enough—and properly aligned, front to back, top to bottom—the adult teeth sometimes could even have the chance, in the growing child, to come in fairly straight all by themselves (or maybe with just a *little* extra help from metal braces, if need be). All of which provide the natural basis for the foundations of a beautiful face.

Consider this: How did all those people out there—and there are millions—who have perfect (or nearly perfect) teeth accomplish a normal-looking (and functioning) bite all by themselves, without any orthodontic help? Answer: They did so because Nature is programmed to develop a human bite that fits that way. There's a word for it: "normal." "Normal" is normal because it's the way things are *supposed* to turn out! Do you ever routinely see a person with one arm or leg substantially longer than the other? Or one eye or one ear several inches higher than the other? Of course not. Nature knows (via the directives of its own genetic code) how to grow the human body correctly. Malocclusions of crooked teeth and/or misaligned jaws don't just happen by accident. Nature knows how to get things right.

Major malocclusions of crooked teeth and misaligned jaws occur because something interferes, forcing the jaws and their passenger teeth to become distorted. Most often the teeth are mere victims in all of this; they get left "holding the orthodontic bag" by virtue of being forced to exhibit the final, crooked result. The true culprit is some type of improperly acting biological force. Many times (though not always) that perpetrator is the imbalanced, overpowering perpetual forces of the surrounding jaw muscles, which, for one reason or another, aren't properly behaving themselves. The Europeans were big on this, and they attempted to develop different ways of straightening out specific skeletal jawbone/muscle distortions that often were responsible for bad bites. They tried to attack the problem at its source—and they did a heck of a job of it. They figured out how to get the jaw muscles "straight" and working right. It seemed like a miracle.

The reason the Europeans believed they could change the "crooked muscle leg" and, as a result, the "crooked bone leg" of the three-legged teeth-bone-muscle maxillofacial triangle was because they actually did it. And they hadn't even meant to. It happened quite by accident.

It all started over a hundred years ago, with a dentist named Viggo Andresen. He was a jovial, bearded, white-haired man who could've been a relative of Santa Claus (though Andresen's beard was much shorter). Originally from Denmark, he moved around Europe and finally wound up in Oslo, Norway, where he practiced both general dentistry and the fledgling science of orthodontics (in the early 1900s, little was yet known about braces).

Dr. Andresen had a daughter who, as a young child, constantly was losing her upper and lower removable orthodontic retainers. So Dr. Andresen decided to glue them together, fashioning one big retainer that would fit at once against both the upper and lower dental arches. Because of its size, it would be more difficult to expel from the little girl's mouth. She wore this device 10-14 hours per day.

But when Dr. Andresen glued the two retainers together, he must not have gotten the upper and lower halves lined up quite right because something incredible happened. Over a period of about nine months of constant wear, this double retainer exerted some strange, mysterious forces on the little girl's jawbones. She'd originally possessed a Skeletal Class II mandibular retrusion (a bite with the undersized lower jaw aligned too far back), but, after utilizing Dr. Andresen's homemade retainer, her mandible was now converted to a full blooming, normally advanced skeletal Class I! It seemed miraculous. (Later, some of these early prototypes of removable, one-piece realigning appliances even picked up the nickname "miracle appliances," because they did what was, up until then, thought to be impossible.) Andresen figured he'd stumbled onto something remarkable. And he had.

A handmade removable orthodontic device could be fabricated—made on plaster replicas of the child's upper and lower teeth—in such a way so as to alter the direction of pull from those bad muscle forces that surrounded the growing jaws. By changing those improper forces, such a device eventually could orchestrate proper jaw size and alignment once more. The trouble was figuring out exactly how it worked. It took not only Dr. Andresen but numerous other prominent dentists across Europe to do so, over a span of 50 years. Plenty of arguments, as you can imagine, were had. But with a great deal of timely help from a wide array of dental professionals, they finally got it worked out.

The technique was given the name *functional jaw orthopedics*, to denote the bone-changing aspects of the method. The removable handmade devices were referred to as *functional appliances* (because the functioning of the jaw muscles around these retainer-like appliances is what made them work). And thus, *functional appliance therapy* in orthodontics was born. Crooked jawbones and crooked-working jaw muscles could now be (somewhat) straightened along with their related teeth. These removable functional appliances were designed to fit comfortably in the mouth. They were also prescribed for wear for the better part of the day and during sleep at night. Being totally removable by the patient (for practical reasons such as eating, active sports, etc.) was another big asset. The metal braces were now used as tooth positioning "perfectors." A better and more biologically comprehensive way had been developed.

Hallelujah!

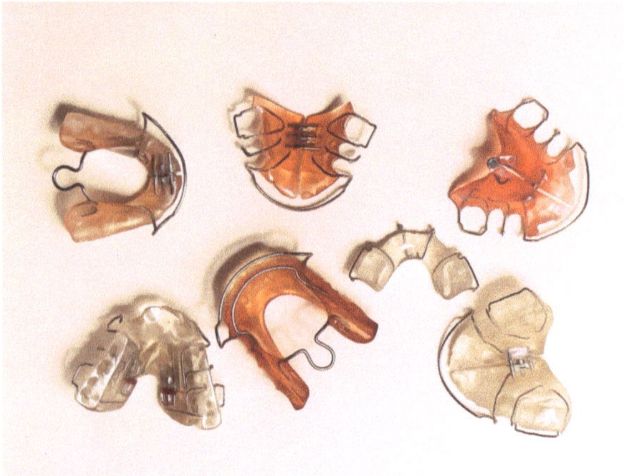

(A)

→ Figure 4-2 (A): Pictured here are a variety of removable functional appliances (the muscle and upper jaw to lower jaw "straighteners" and "jaw socket fixers") as well as a few of the equally removable *active plates* (bone and teeth "shapers") that are currently in use within modern orthodontic treatment. Often, old-fashioned metal braces are used in conjunction with, or in addition to, removable functional appliances in a comprehensive treatment plan for severe malocclusions. Metal braces are still the best tool for twisting, leveling, or angulating individual crooked teeth.

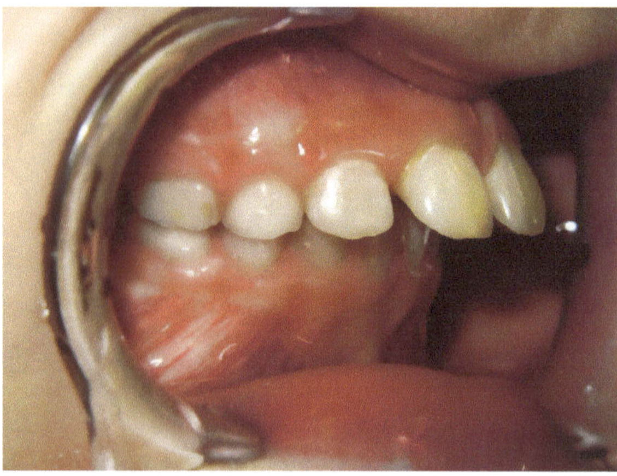

(B)

→ Figure 4-2 (B): Here is a starting picture of a nine-year-old girl with a typical Class II malocclusion in which the upper teeth appear to be out too far. At this age, the child's teeth are in what we call the *mixed dentition*, which means permanent teeth have come in (or *erupted*, as dentists say) in the front and the back, but, in between, the deciduous (or baby) teeth haven't fallen out yet. These types of cases were once treated by retracting the upper front teeth back with metal braces (and maybe even extracting upper bicuspids, one on each side, to aid the retraction) in order to meet the lowers. This often left the finished facial profile and lower jaw line retruded. Not good!

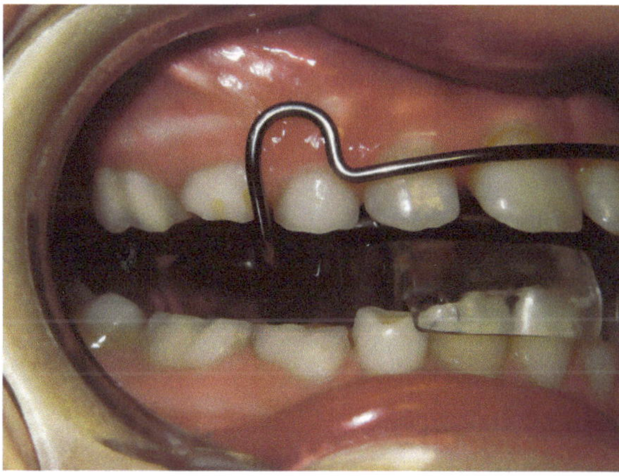

(C)

→ Figure 4-2 (C): A patient wearing a functional appliance called a Bionator, which helps correct the malocclusion (a severe Class II). The child wore the Bionator during the day, but nonstop during the evening and through the night. Remember: Functional appliances are removeable by the patient and can be used in the mixed dentition because they don't attach to the teeth like metal braces do. Generally, you don't put metal braces on baby teeth; dentists like to wait until all of them fall out and the new adult teeth come in. In the meantime, the child's malocclusion often keeps collapsing (and, usually, the face along with it).

(Continued)

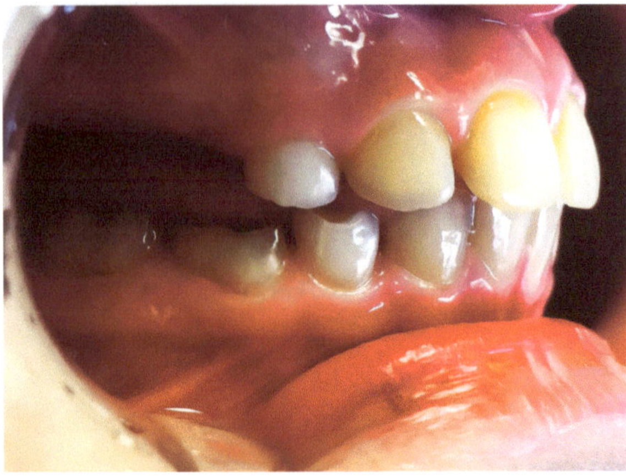

(D)

→ Figure 4-2 (D): The nine-year-old patient after nine months of treatment with the Bionator (worn mostly at night during sleep and only partially during the day). Notice how some of the upper baby teeth have fallen out, but, because the appliance is removable and not attached to any teeth (like metal braces), treatment with the Bionator may continue, even as doctor and patient await the remainder of the permanent teeth, which often take months or even several years to erupt. (When those permanent teeth *do* break through the gums, the design of the Bionator will guide them into a perfect final position.) Also observe how the lower jaw has come permanently forward as well as how the lower front teeth show more prominently—as they're supposed to—compared to how hidden they were in the pre-treatment bite. Dentists call this process "increasing the vertical dimension of occlusion," which helps fill out the lower facial profile to its normal proportions, thus increasing overall facial beauty. Two great things!

Functional appliances were first used here during the '60s and '70s. Instead of employing the more modern, streamlined, high-powered version of the appliances that were just then being perfected in Europe, American researchers conducted preliminary studies on patients with several of the early prototypes (for example, one called The Activator), which were more primitive and far less efficient. Furthermore, they didn't really use the devices all that well—owing to a lack of understanding regarding important construction and management details—and so, they generally got poor results.

They blamed this failure on the appliances themselves rather than on their own shortcomings. When initial experimental studies were complete, American orthodontic researchers and university professors published findings that said the treatment results were not very promising. They just couldn't seem to get the same kind of increased jawbone growth and forward-realignment results the Europeans were talking about.

Much of the orthodontic community in America took these experimenters' word at face value and didn't bother to do the homework for themselves. Consequently, as removable functional appliances were reaching their zenith in Europe during the '70s, '80s, and '90s, they still were being viewed here in America by the initial standards by which they were first judged.

But guess what? New, definitive studies have since been published on the performance of the newer designs, showcasing their effectiveness. Today's version of these removable functional appliances are now made with more modern materials such as lightweight but strong dental acrylic instead of the old bulky vulcanite (the same hard, rubbery material they use to make hockey pucks!) from some 80 years ago. And now the real verdict is finally in, and it is indisputable: Functional appliances work!

And not only do they work, they work spectacularly well, just like the old-time European dentists said they would. The secret lies in knowing just how—and when—to use them. Once you know that, the rest is easy!

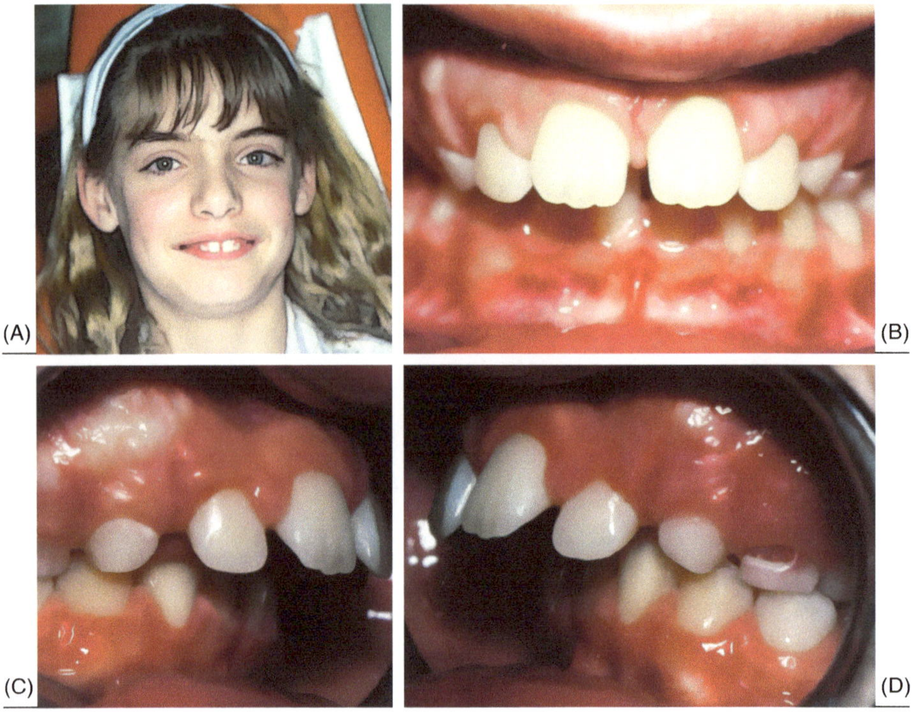

→ Figures 4-3 (A - D): Here is a picture of a pretty young girl, but she appears (notice I used the word *appears*) to be suffering from "buck teeth" and an upper front jaw that is sticking out too far. Not so! Appearances like this are actually most often due to the whole lower jaw being back too far.

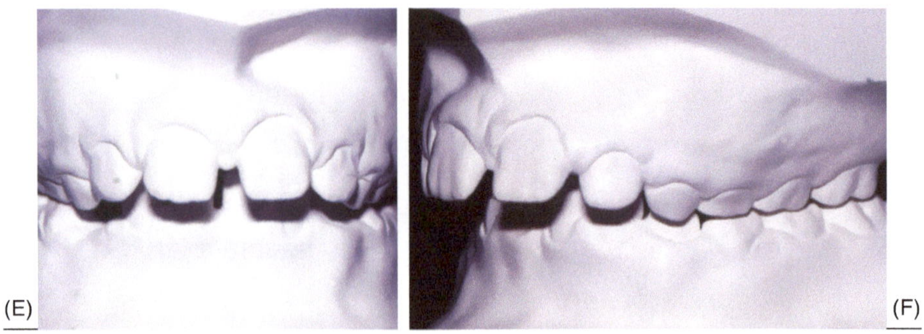

→ Figures 4-3 (E, F): White plaster models (dentists call them *study casts*) that demonstrate the patient's malocclusion. The upper jawbone itself is also too narrow.

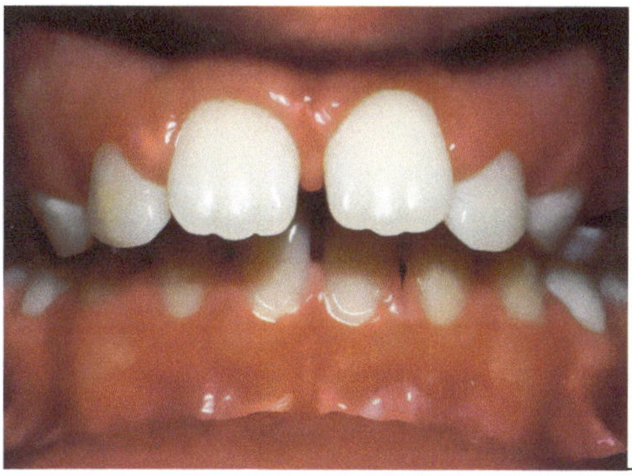
(G)

→ Figure 4-3 (G): The pre-treatment *intra-oral* (or inside the mouth) photograph of the child's malocclusion.

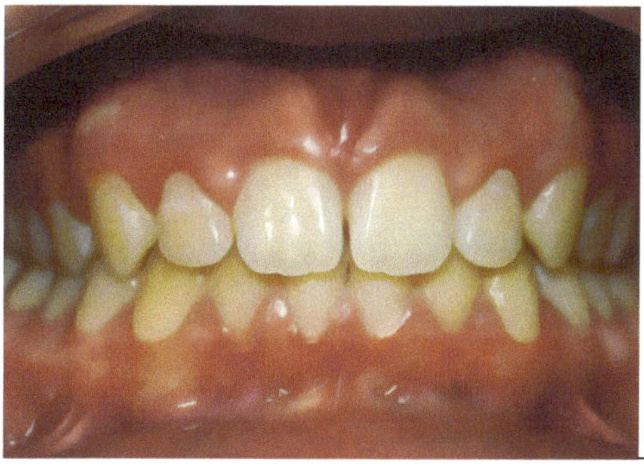
(H)

→ Figure 4-3 (H): Figure 4-3 (G) stands in stark contrast to this image, which shows the post-treatment intra-oral photograph of the finished case, treated almost exclusively with removable functional appliances. The retruded lower jaw and its teeth were brought forward (permanently) to properly align with the correctly positioned upper jaw and teeth.

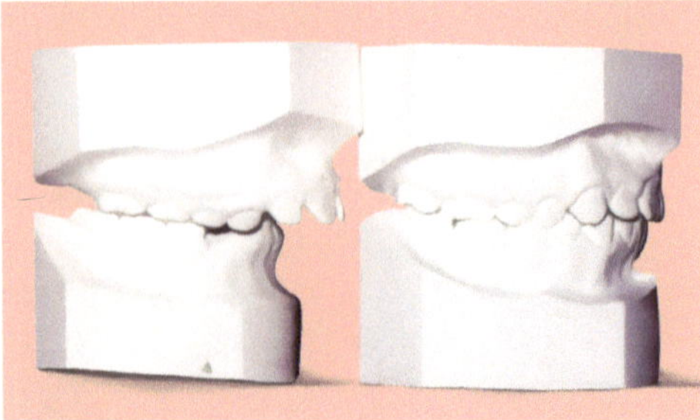

(I)

→ Figure 4-3 (I): A right-side view of both the pre-treatment and post-treatment study casts for this patient.

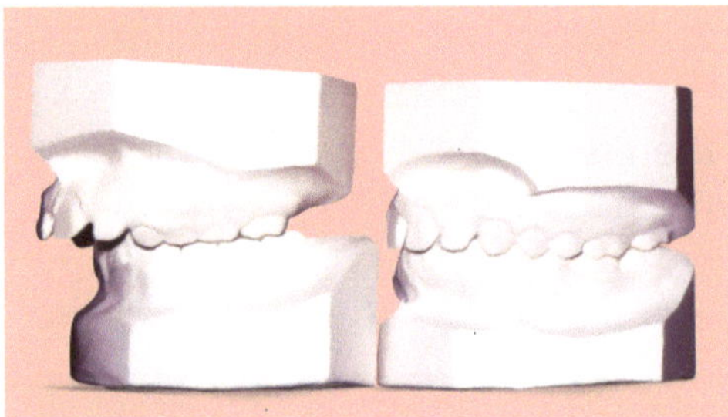

(J)

→ Figure 4-3 (J): A left-side view of both the pre-treatment and post-treatment study casts. Again, the lower jaw was brought forward to meet the upper, *not* vice versa.

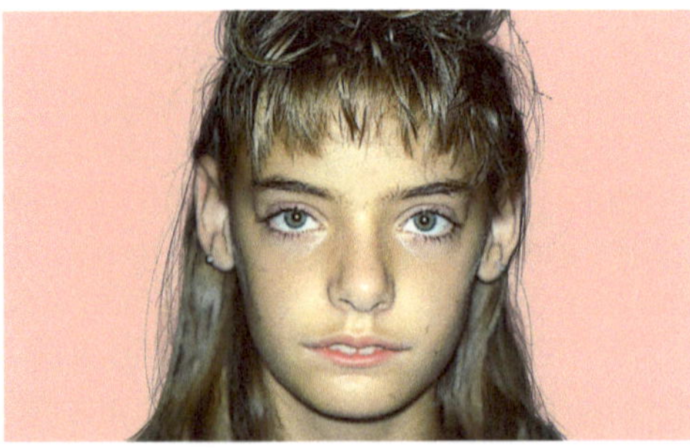

(K)

→ Figure 4-3 (K): A pre-treatment frontal image (note the recessed lower jaw and prominent upper front teeth protruding between the lips).

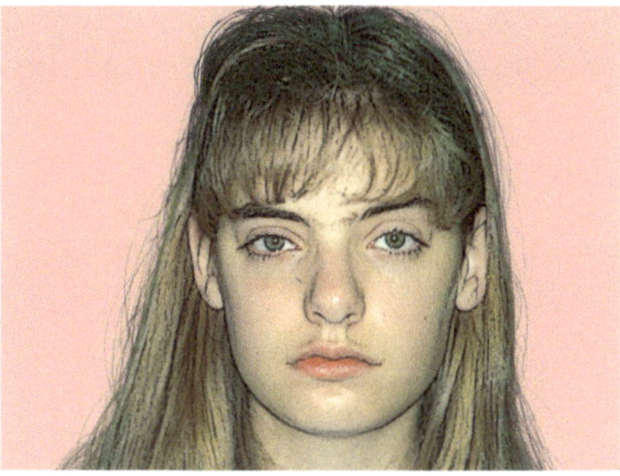

(L)

→ Figure 4-3 (L): A post-treatment frontal image. As they say, *Res ipsa loquitur* (Latin for "The thing speaks for itself").

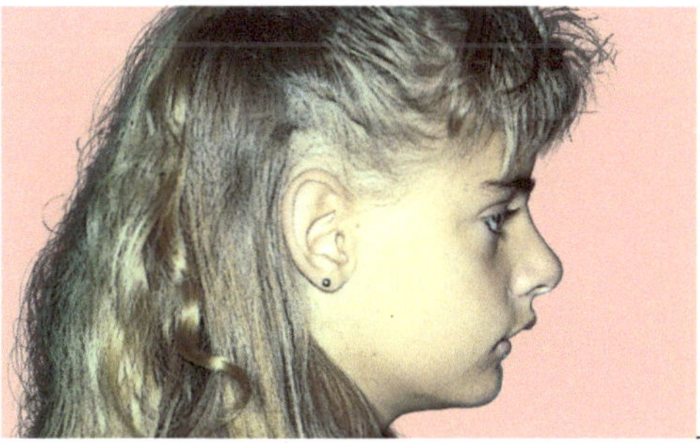

(M)

→ Figure 4-3 (M): The pre-treatment retruded lower facial profile.

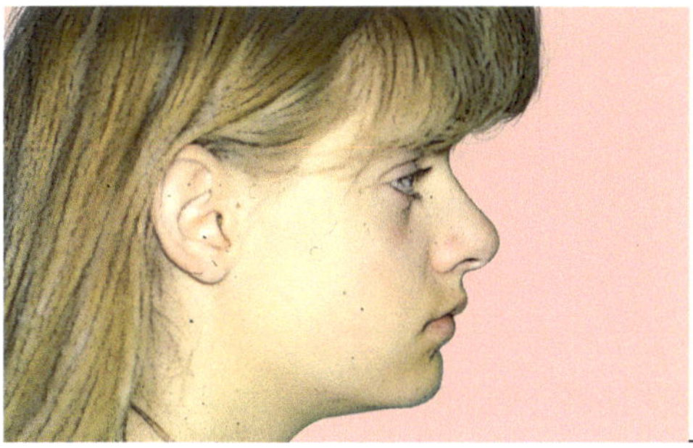

(N)

→ Figure 4-3 (N): The post-treatment filled-out facial profile thanks to removable functional appliances. (Note: A few months of metal braces also were used to perfect individual *tooth angulation* and apply some minor finishing touches. Very little was needed. Nothing beats traditional metal braces for precise tooth positioning and *tooth root angulation.*)

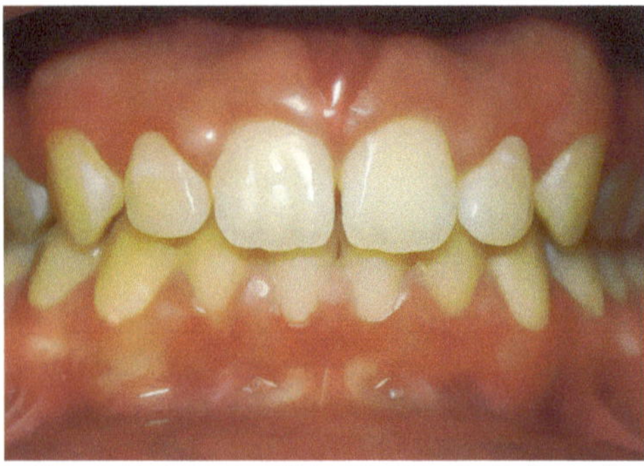

(O)

→ Figure 4-3 (O): The final occlusion. This is in the proper fit of both the teeth *and* the jaws.

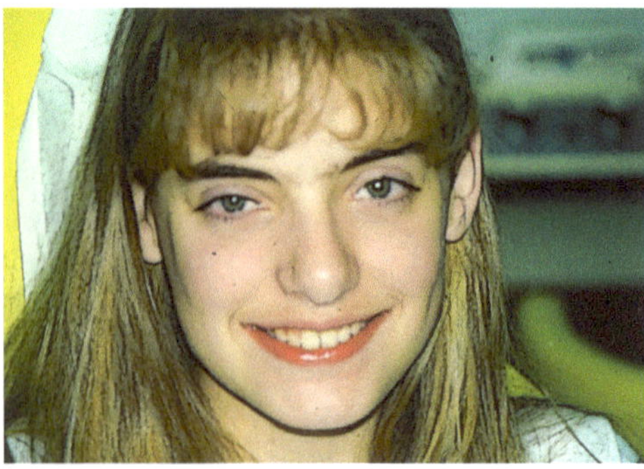

(P)

→ Figure 4-3 (P): A final picture of the now-beautiful young woman. Functional appliances: the plastic fantastic!

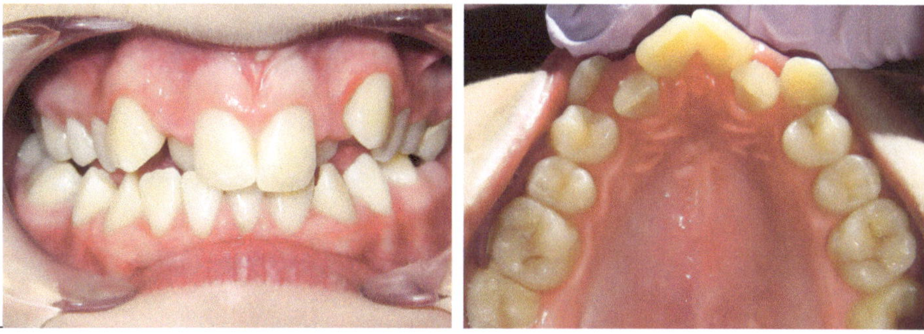

(A) (B)

→ Figures 4-4 (A, B): Here are some images of another pretty young girl—but, alas, her teeth require a little help. Notice how gothic, triangular, and arrowhead-shaped her upper jawbone is. This results in tremendous jumbling and crowding in the upper front teeth. Straightening these teeth within such an undersized and deformed upper jaw is very difficult, if not impossible, without bilaterally extracting permanent adult teeth, one per side, to shoehorn in the remaining teeth with a reasonably straight appearance.

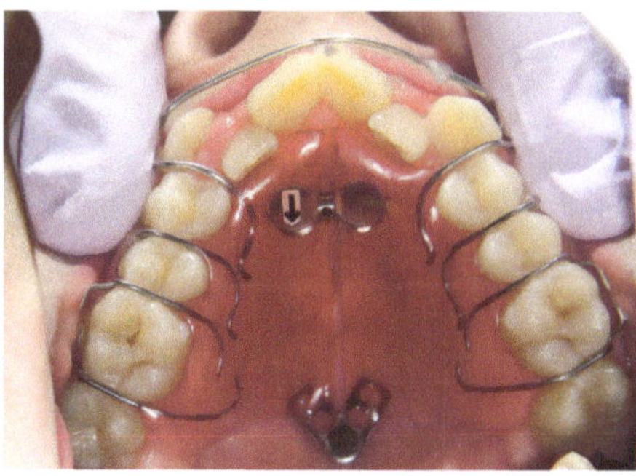

(C)

→ Figure 4-4 (C): Enter active plates, first cousins to functional appliances. These types of removable appliances are famous for being powerful bone movers and bone re-shapers, just what is needed here. After about four months of incremental activation (performed biweekly, and at home by the patient), this first appliance resulted in a bigger, wider, more Roman arch-shaped appearance to the front part of the upper arch.

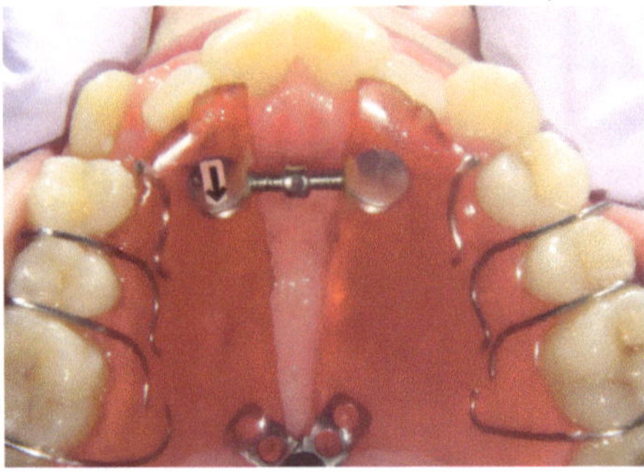

(D)

→ Figure 4-4 (D): Since a special little *active expansion screw* in the appliance only opens so far, a new second appliance was needed (what's called a *FAN appliance*, for obvious reasons). This supplemental device was constructed to fit the newly shaped dental arch, and it was used to continue making the upper jaw wider and more Roman-arched.

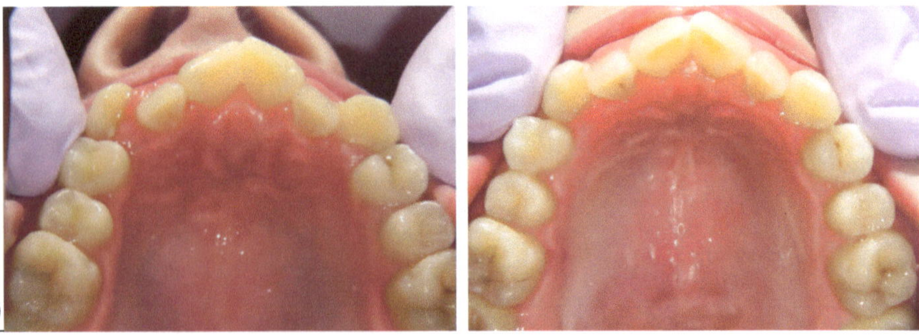

(E) (F)

→ Figures 4-4 (E, F): Bone-moving improvements complete! Observe how far the passenger upper teeth have traveled (straightening out on their own as part of the process). Now, there is plenty of room to straighten those teeth that last little bit using traditional metal braces. The jawbones themselves can now accommodate all those teeth without the necessity of extracting any of them—i.e., all the teeth can be made to fit naturally, the way Mother Nature intended.

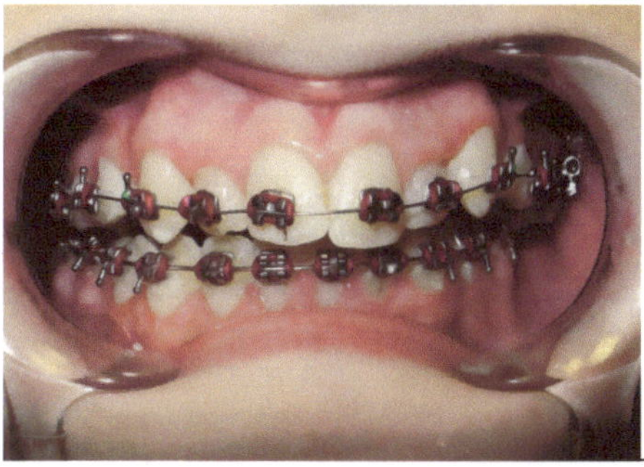

(G)

→ Figure 4-4 (G): Metal braces were applied for about six months to perfect the individual tooth positioning and angulation. (One of the oldest rules in orthodontics states that, "First you must have the actual space ... then you must have some bone in that space in order to move a tooth *into* that space!")

(H)

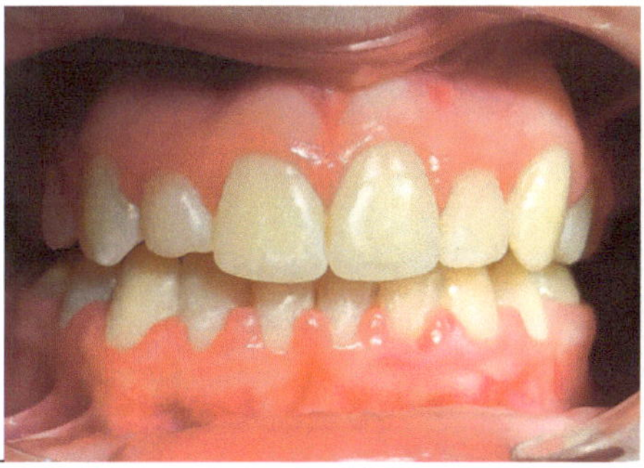

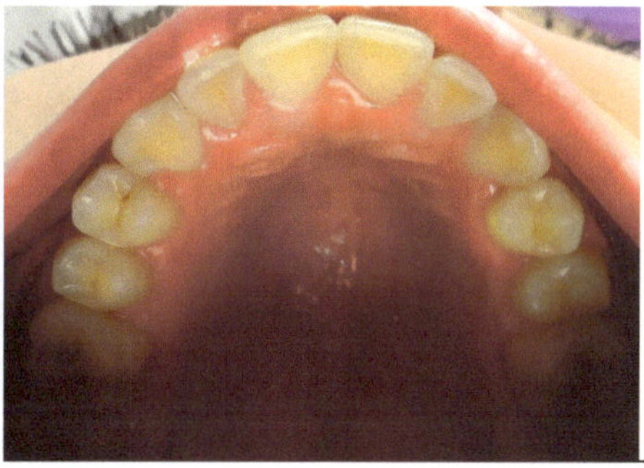

(I)

→ Figures 4-4 (H, I): The finished product (compare to Figures 4-4 (A, B). Notice all of the teeth are present (non-extraction) in a properly sized—and properly shaped—upper jawbone, which was made bigger and properly formed to hold all the teeth. (The alternative would have been to make the remaining teeth [after extraction] fit into a smaller jaw that was improperly sized.)

(Continued)

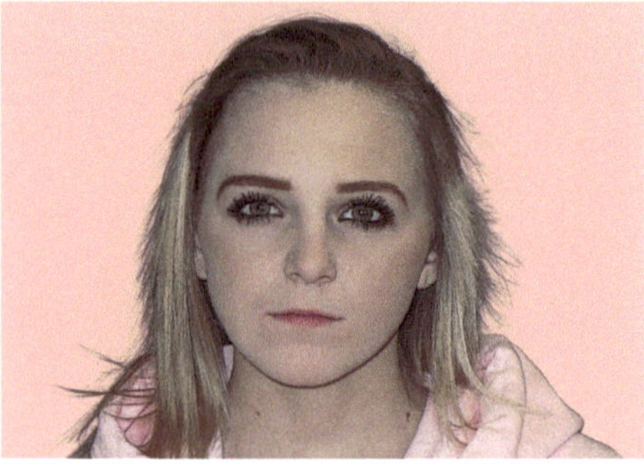

(J)

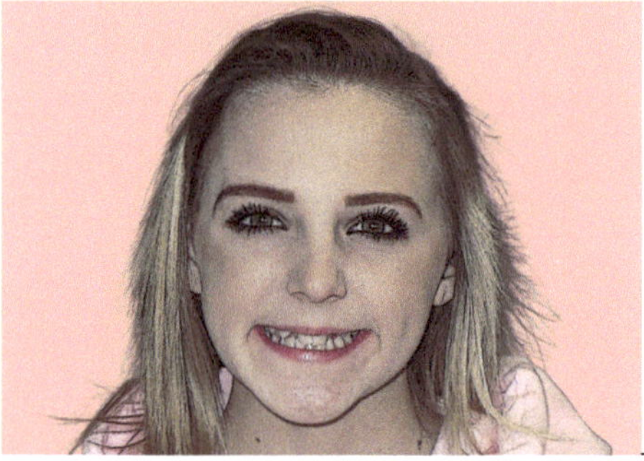

(K)

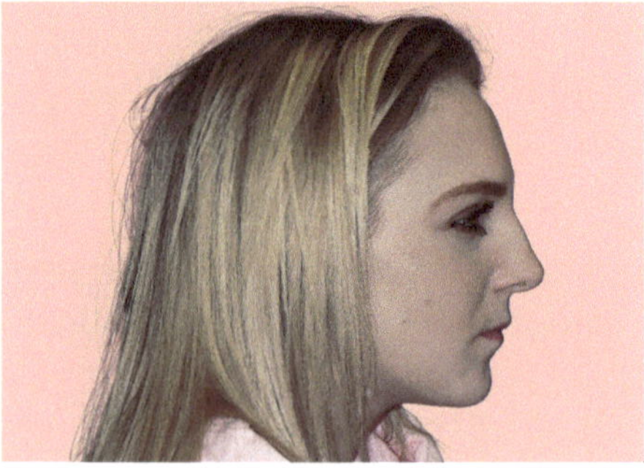

(L)

→ Figures 4-4 (J - L): Frontal and profile facial appearance, pre-treatment, of the patient in the preceding images (Figure 4-4 [A] to Figure 4-4 [I]). Notice the somewhat retruded lower profile of the jawline.

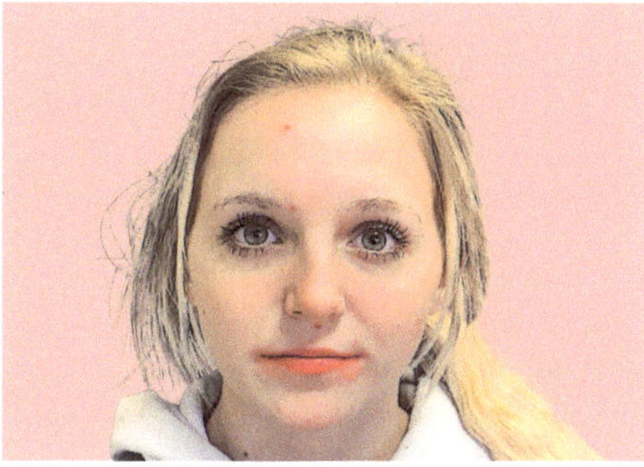

(M)

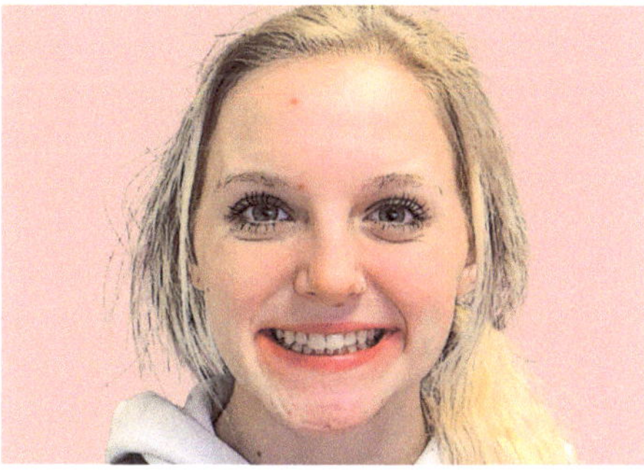

(N)

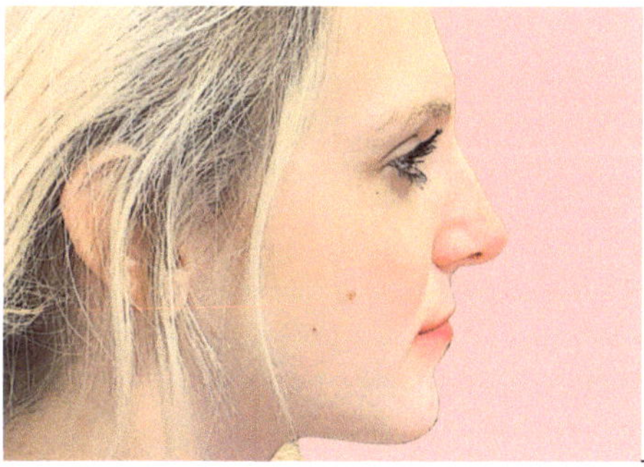

(O)

→ Figures 4-4 (M - O): Frontal and profile facial appearance, post-treatment. Notice the improved profile of the now correctly positioned lower jaw, which was relocated via other conventional functional orthopedic techniques (all of which were part of the overall treatment plan, but are not pictured here).

Figure 4-4 (P)

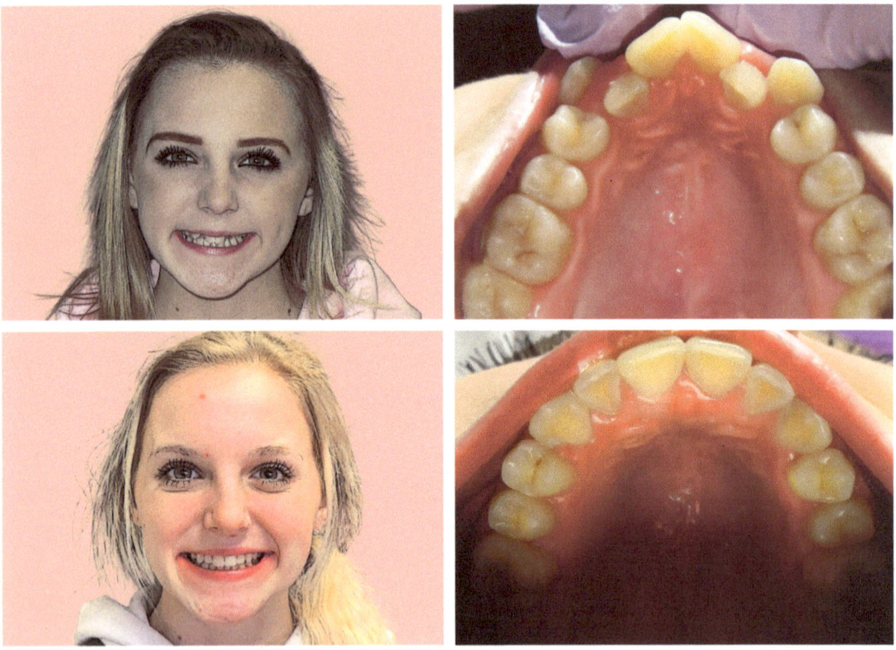

→ A side-by-side comparison of the pre- and post-treatment facial appearance as well as the upper dental arch. As you can see: In this case, functional jaw orthopedic techniques were the way to go! (A side note: Before treatment, this patient suffered from dysfunctional jaw joint clicking, especially upon chewing; sore jaw joints and facial muscles; and repeated headaches. After treatment, these signs and symptoms disappeared. She remains headache- and facial pain-free to this day.)

FIVE

Extractions Revisited: Second Thoughts

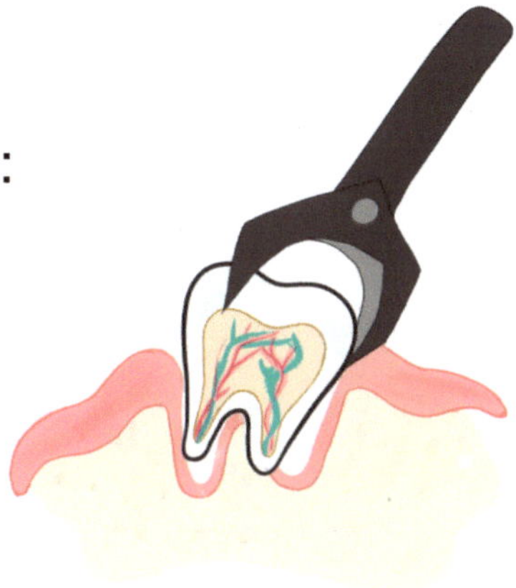

It is difficult suddenly to lay aside a long-cherished love.

— Catullus (84-54 B.C),
Roman poet

I know it seems like I'm piling on yet more material to an already complex—and confusing—subject, but true empowerment for the layperson comes from complete knowledge of the "ins-and-outs." And one of the most important concerns is which permanent teeth are kept, and which are removed. It's really not too difficult to understand, so stick with me on this. It's important stuff.

We have seen now, from an orthopedic standpoint, how the ability of European-style removable functional orthodontic acrylic appliances has created an enormous dichotomy in the approach to treating the common Class II malocclusion (under-developed lower jaw). On one side, we have the traditional American school of thought, which generally forces the upper dental arch and upper front teeth backward to meet the lower teeth in the retruded lower jaw. On the other side of this controversy lies the newer European approach, which essentially leaves the upper arch and upper teeth where they are but brings the entire retruded lower jaw forward to meet the stationary upper jaw. The Americans said, in effect, forcing retruded, misaligned lower jaws in children to grow out forward couldn't be done—i.e., the kid was "deformed" jaw-wise and would just have to live with it. The Europeans, on the other hand, said realigning the lower jaw correctly forward *could* be done—and had proven it. Despite all this, the fight between the two viewpoints waged for decades and, in some circles, incredibly, still continues to this day!

But there's more. As if things weren't already hot enough between the American-fixed-appliance (metal braces only) school of thought and the European removable-functional-appliance approach (in conjunction with metal braces), things get really heated when it comes to the revolutionary way in which Europeans address the problem of dental extractions. Some malocclusions are so severe that certain permanent teeth do, in fact, need to be extracted in children and/or adults for the sake of creating enough room to straighten and unjumble the remaining teeth, thereby helping the braces work. But the Europeans—and a few forward-thinking Americans—figured out how to do it in a whole new way. A better way.

Now, using removable acrylic intra-oral functional appliances to change and correct the aberrant surrounding oral muscle environment—and thereby gradually correct the entire misaligned lower jaw—is all fine and good, but it still doesn't do much to solve the problem of lining up crooked, jammed, or crowded teeth. That process still requires some form of a more traditional, forceful, tooth-directed, metal brace–type approach. But applying those forces and straightening everything out is all but impossible—regardless of what type of brace system you use—unless you have the room in the jaws to do it.

The Europeans realized this and accepted the fact that, yes, there *are* times when the dental arches of individual teeth have collapsed so badly and the teeth themselves have become so crooked or overlapped and otherwise displaced that the only way you can move those teeth far enough apart to straighten them out is to sacrifice a few of them by means of purposeful extraction. Thus, sometimes extracting bicuspids *is* the right thing to do. But not always. In an even larger number of cases, it simply isn't. The extraction of the bicuspids is fraught with all sorts of potential long-term problems, manifested in the patient's final facial aesthetics as well as in other technical issues of an orthopedic nature.

So, years ago, a search was begun by forward-thinking dentists who were determined to discover a solution to the orthodontic dental crowding/extraction problem. As it turned out, the answer emerged—almost simultaneously—on both American and European shores. It still involved extracting permanent adult teeth, but instead of targeting the bicuspids in the front of the dental arches by the corners of the mouth, it advised the clever notion of extracting 12-year (or second) molars from the back. This radical new method was looked upon by the Europeans—and an increasing number of more modern-thinking American converts—as a miraculous stroke of genius, one capable of solving the staggering problems inherent within the dental extraction process (but only for adolescent patients). In contrast, the technique of choosing different teeth to extract was viewed, at least at first, as incomprehensible malpractice by many in the United States, especially orthodontic traditionalists. It left them totally aghast. But again, the Europeans turned out to be right. Here's why.

Over time, dental clinicians discovered that, if timed properly during the adolescent and teenage years—when the third molars are present but still unerupted, developing in their respective bony sockets below the gums—the extraction of the second molars (for any reason) can, in effect, "wake up" the wisdom teeth. Thus roused, the third molars often will be stimulated to grow and move in, two to five years earlier than normal, directly into the space once occupied by the extracted second molars (or, right behind the remaining first molars). In each of the four quadrants, then, you will see two bicuspids and two molars, the first and the third. When all is said and done, the back of the mouth will appear just like a normal adult dentition—as if nothing had happened!

In the meantime, all the orthodontic "unjumbling" of the other crowded teeth will easily be completed, made possible by the newly created space at the second-molar extraction site. This technique preserves the full size and width of the front dental arch, as the bicuspids aren't extracted in the old, traditional method, allowing for a smile that is much fuller and, hence, more attractive!

For many years, there has been a misconception among laypeople regarding wisdom teeth: that they are not as "good" as their fellows because they're weaker or have poor enamel. Friends, this is false! They *are* just as good as any other tooth. Like fingernails, ribs, or eyelashes, one is about the same as the next.

There also is a common misconception among dental professionals that wisdom teeth often develop their roots improperly in their bony sockets, in a twisted fashion. False again. Third molar wisdom teeth can develop curved, hooked, or otherwise crooked roots as the tooth is forming down within its *embryonic sac* while still in the jawbone. But there is a reason this sometimes—and *only* sometimes—occurs. All the other teeth have plenty of room within their sockets for their roots to grow normally. The poor last set of third molars, however, are sometimes forced to contort their developing roots in deformed and strange manners because, as they develop, the wisdom teeth are most often physically cramped by the back angle of the jaw. But if those wisdom teeth are given enough room to maneuver—i.e., to grow and erupt properly—then their roots will also form correctly, just like the other teeth.

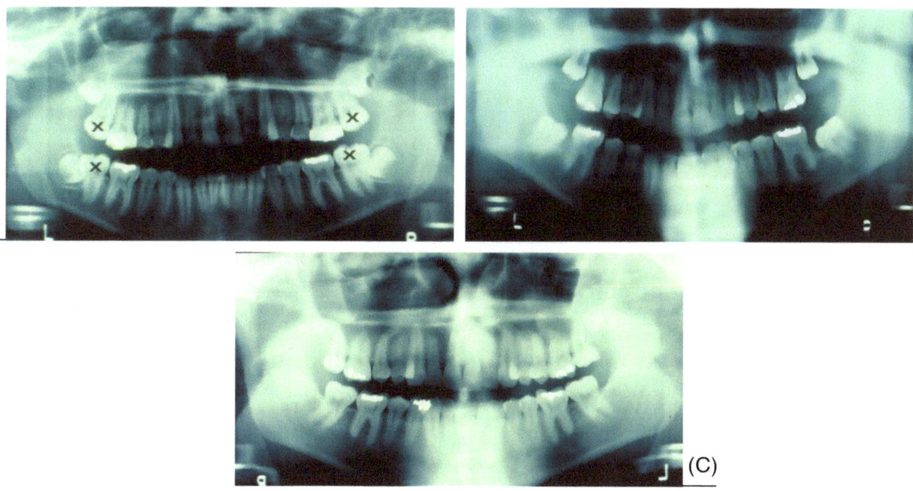

(A) (B) (C)

→ Figures 5-1 (A - C): Here are a series of X-rays called *orthopantomograms* (also known as *pantographs* or the abbreviated *pans*). This type of X-ray takes the human jaws—which are essentially spherical (or round in three dimensions)—and flattens them out in the form of a two-dimensional image. This allows the entire upper and lower jaws (as well as their passenger teeth) to be seen simultaneously, in one image.

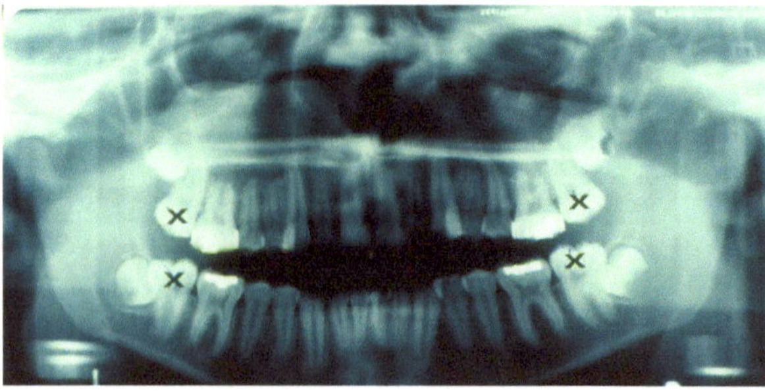

(A)

→ Figure 5-1 (A): In this first pre-treatment image of a 14-year-old boy, the four second molars (teeth with the *X's* on them) have been slated for removal due to specific treatment planning reasons.

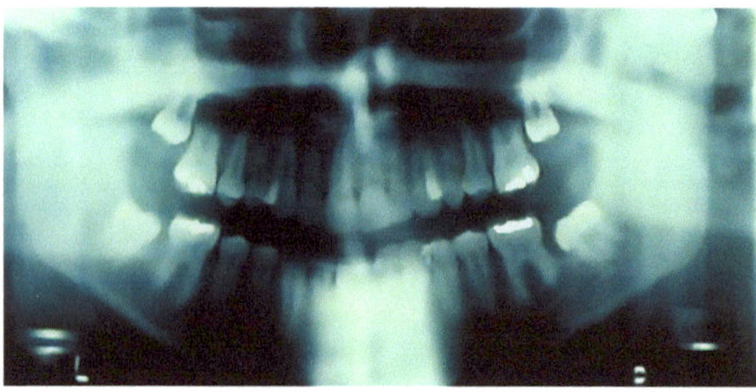

(B)

→ Figure 5-1 (B): In this image, taken several years later, all four second molars have been removed, and the socket bone where they were located has healed back in. You can also see that the third molars (or the wisdom teeth) have developed more rapidly than usual and are in the process of moving into the spaces formerly occupied by the extracted second molars. In the interim the jumbled, crooked teeth have been orthodontically straightened much more easily, bicuspids and all, because of the extra space provided for them in the perimeter and back of the dental arches by the vacated second molar extraction sites.

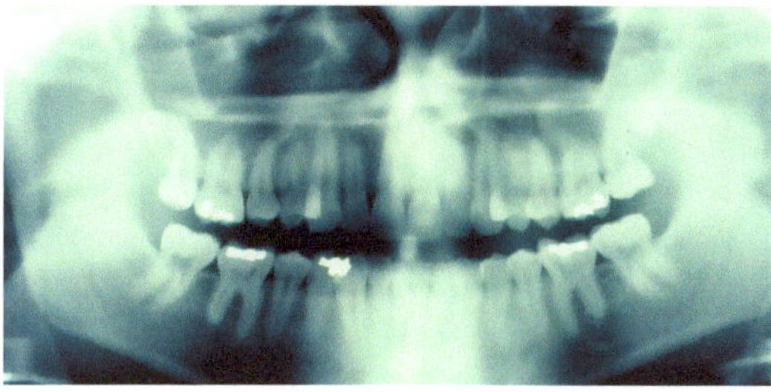

(C)

→ Figure 5-1 (C): The finished result, several years later. No difficult third molar surgery needed here!

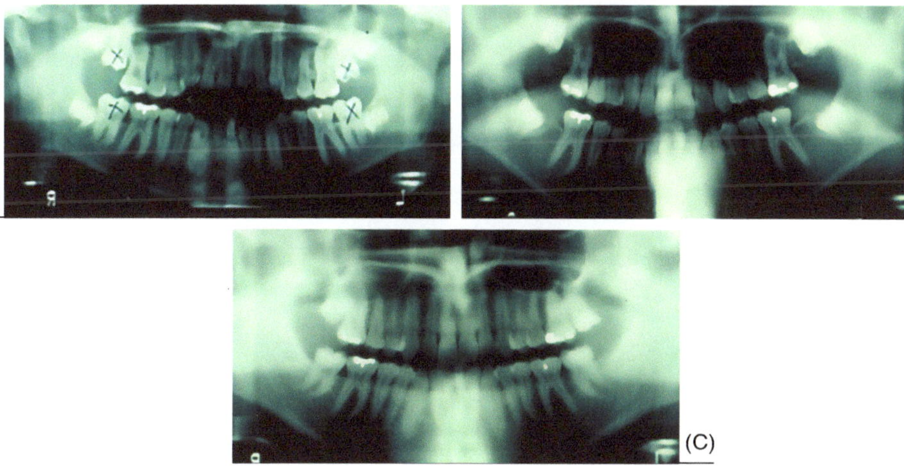

(A) (B) (C)

→ Figures 5-2 (A - C): Here are another set of pantographs of a female teenager who underwent a similar, specifically prescribed second molar extraction treatment.

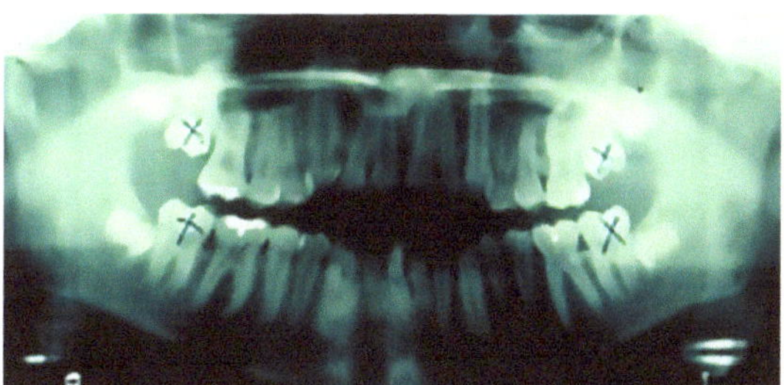

(A)

→ Figure 5-2 (A): A pre-treatment image showing the second molars that will be extracted (marked with *X's*).

Notice the third molars are still developing within their sockets. In fact, their roots haven't even formed yet.

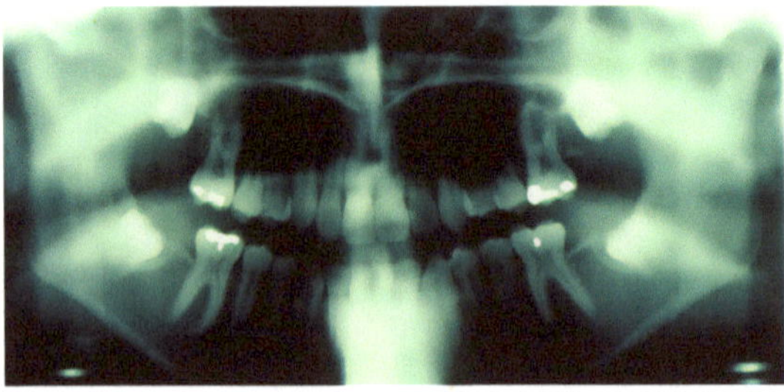

(B)

→ Figure 5-2 (B): An image taken a year and a half later. Notice how, after the second molars have been extracted, the third molars are developing quite nicely—even if they're still relatively distant from the extracted second molar positions.

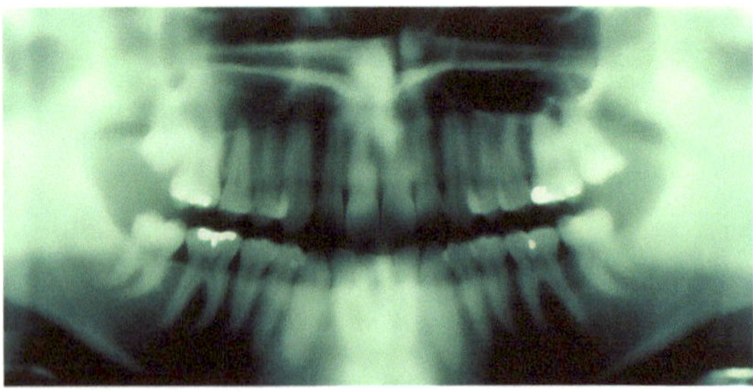

(C)

→ Figure 5-2 (C): The finished result, several years later. No dentist unfamiliar with the history of this case could look at the finished film and tell whether those four backmost teeth are second or third molars (which have, in fact, replaced them).

Special Note: An orthodontic specialist named Dr. James Evans (now retired) is famous for having removed over 20,000 second molars throughout his lengthy career (which featured a tenure as the head of a major Midwestern university's orthodontic department).

Another orthodontic specialist of note is Dr. Johnathan Parker (now deceased). Originally from Monroe, Louisiana, he was a member of the American Board of Orthodontics (ABO), which is a very high honor among our ilk. In order to be elevated to the ABO, candidates must go through rigorous examinations as well as present numerous cases they have treated and finished—all done before a panel of meticulous examiners who comb through every detail, scouring for the slightest fault to gripe about. In the old days, only 23% of orthodontic specialists made it onto the ABO. Dr. Parker, meanwhile, was elevated to that prestigious position by showing nothing other than second molar extraction cases, which he had treated to board-qualifying status! *Every* orthodontist, whether or not they personally agree with this technique, should have at least heard of the procedure. A number of their prestigious colleagues certainly have.

(A) 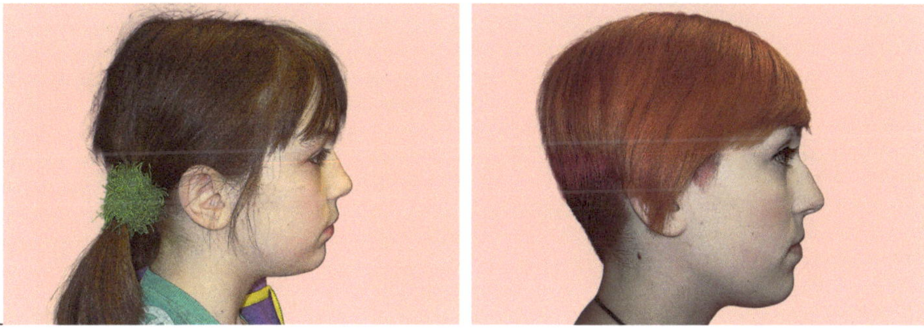 (B)

→ Figures 5-3 (A, B): Pre-treatment vs. post-treatment profiles.

(C) 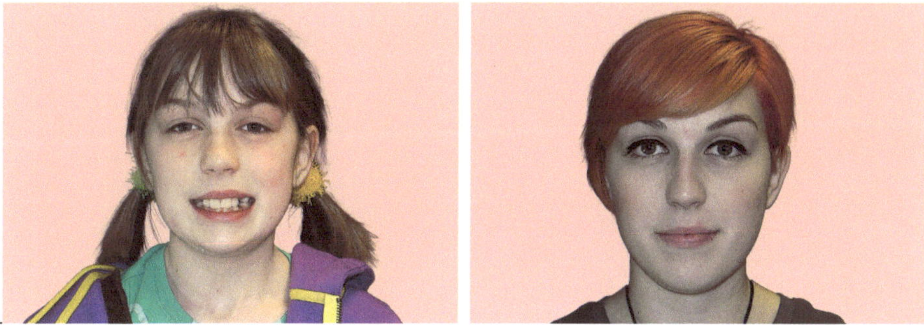 (D)

→ Figures 5-3 (C, D): Pre-treatment vs. post-treatment frontal view of the other patient. Notice, in these first four images, the post-treatment fullness of both the facial profile, lip contours, and the plumpness of the lower jaw and face. Nice!

(Continued)

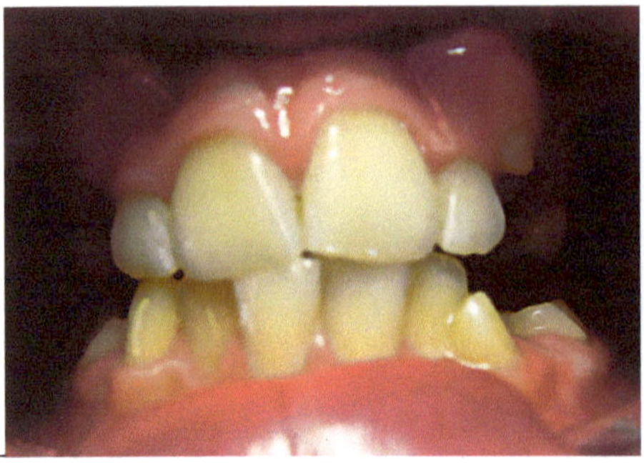
(E)

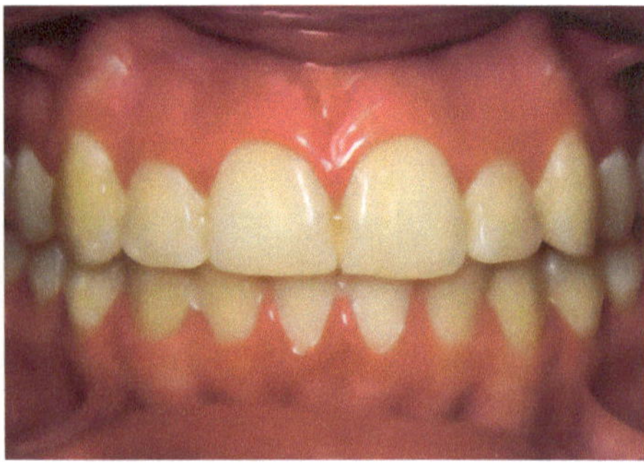
(F)

→ Figures 5-3 (E, F): Pre-treatment vs. post-treatment frontal views. Note: (E) is where the patient liked to rest her lower jaw.

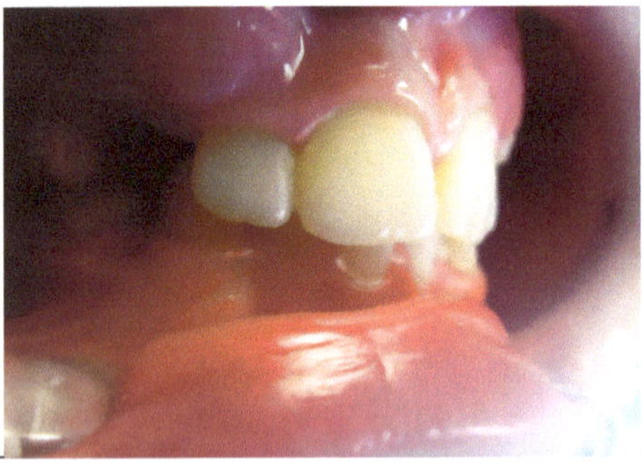
(G)

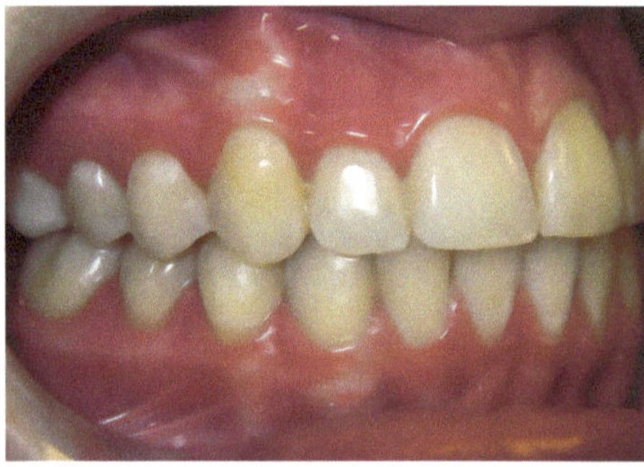
(H)

→ Figures 5-3 (G, H): Pre-treatment vs post-treatment occlusions from the right side. Note: (G) is where the patient actually bit down.

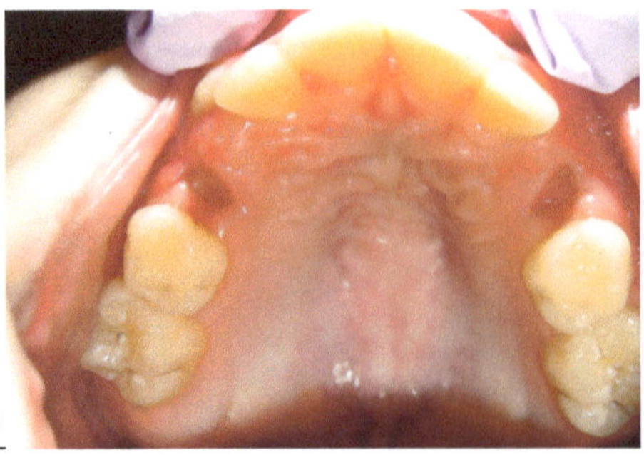
(I)

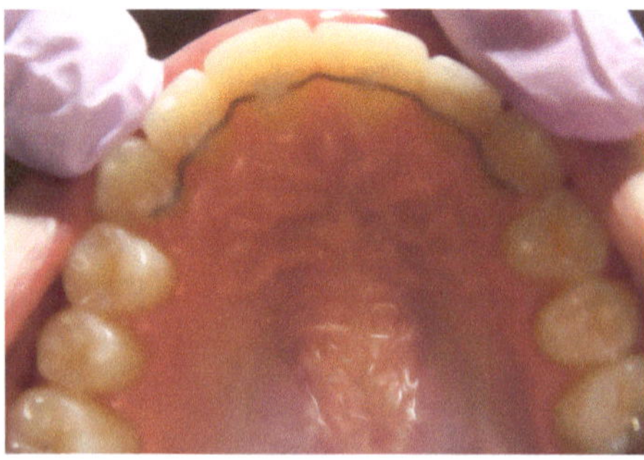
(J)

→ Figures 5-3 (I, J): Pre-treatment vs. post-treatment *occlusal* views of the upper arch. Take note of one important thing: See that gap between the last upper front tooth and the first upper back tooth in the pre-treatment image?

Currently, that space isn't big enough to accommodate the two large adult teeth waiting to erupt. If you look carefully, you can just make out (on the left) one of those upper adult teeth coming in, right on top of the second front tooth. In the post-treatment view, all of the teeth are present except the upper second molars, which have been extracted. Not to worry; the upper third molars are developing in their sockets, just waiting to move into the space formerly occupied by the second molars. Also notice the wire retainer glued to the back sides of the upper front teeth—or, the traditional way to retain these teeth after they've been moved with metal braces. These types of retainers are often still used at the end of treatment. They can remain in place for several years (or longer) depending on need. (Metal braces were used here to "touch up" individual tooth position and angulation—all in conjunction with functional appliance treatments that corrected the bones and muscles.)

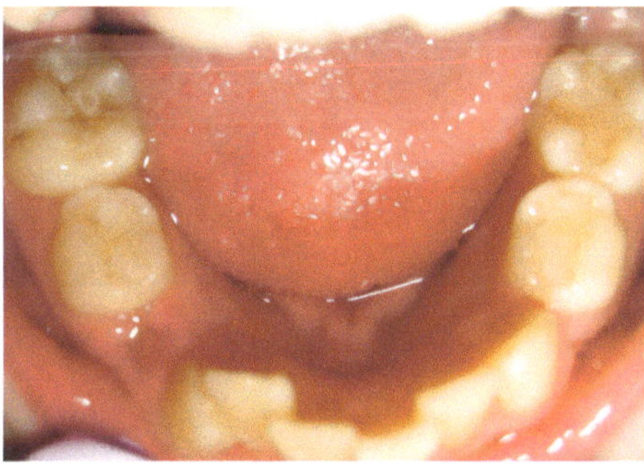

(K)

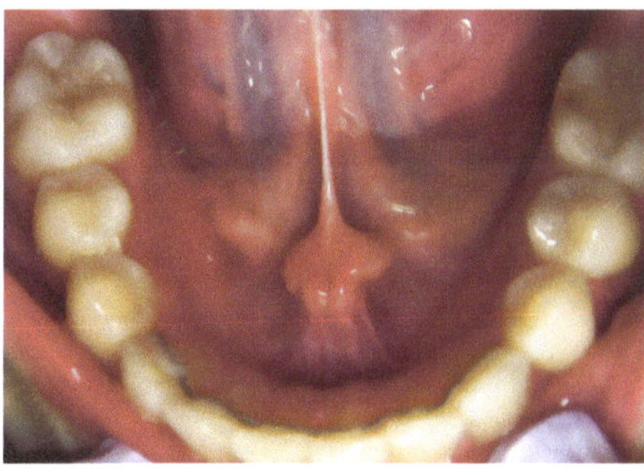

(L)

→ Figures 5-3 (K, L): Pre-treatment vs. post-treatment occlusal view of the lower arch. The same principles seen in Figures 5-3 (I, J) apply.

(Continued)

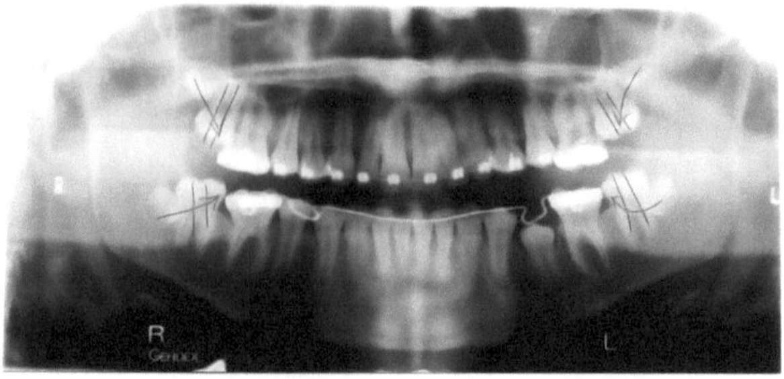

(M)

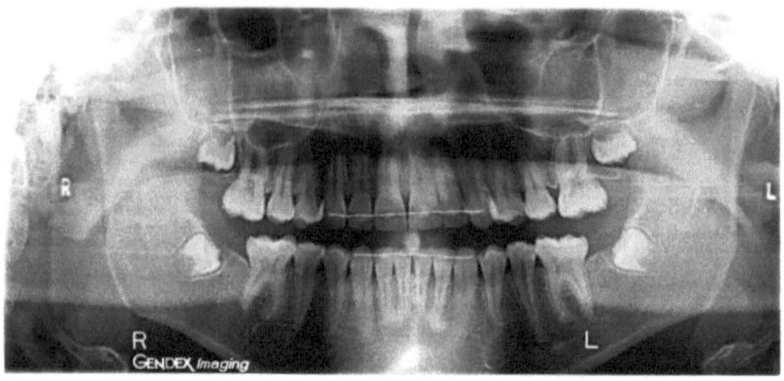

(N)

→ Figures 5-3 (M, N): Pre-treatment (M) and mid-treatment (N) pantographic X-rays showing how the extraction of the four second molars (which greatly facilitated the treatment) has stimulated the third molars into moving forward. They'll eventually erupt into the space once occupied by the second molars. This young girl was diagnosed by means of sophisticated X-ray analysis; she was determined to be exhibiting a Dental, Skeletal, and Condylar Class II malocclusion. This means that, not only was the vertical alignment of the upper and lower teeth off, the jawbones and jaw sockets themselves were also misplaced, with the latter jammed back too far at full bite. That's begging for trouble! But now, thanks to functional orthodontics and functional orthopedic principles of treatment, this patient now exhibits a full Class I-type occlusion—*and* doesn't have headaches!

Note: Extracting second molars (in order to let the third molars replace them) is easier, safer, and far less expensive.

Yes, if you want to split hairs, there *is* a small percentage of wisdom teeth that might be slightly smaller than the normal second molars they would be replacing. So what? Big deal! It's not an arm or a leg. A slightly smaller tooth in the back of your mouth often beats the final appearance that results from the traditional orthodontic tooth extraction method, which can lead to a caved-in face, a sunken smile, and, most gravely, a self-conscious adolescent personality. (See the "Eirew twins.")

As an experiment, ask your son or daughter which option they would prefer. If forced to undergo one extraction technique or another, would they rather have a treatment that would result in 1) a full, rounded-out face and a broad, symmetrical smile, but the last tooth in the back of the mouth would be a third molar instead of a second in each of the four quadrants—and, thus, possibly a little smaller; *or*, 2) the possibility of a flattened smile line with a narrower, less full-looking set of teeth as well as a lower jaw/chin that might look retruded and underdeveloped (but the last tooth in each quadrant would be the usual, larger second molar)?

Furthermore, your son or daughter would, in option two, most likely still need all four of their third molars surgically extracted the old way (and, lest you forget, extracting wisdom teeth can be an arduous and painful procedure). In summary, it's a matter of only four teeth extracted the new way, versus a total of eight teeth extracted through the traditional style.

It doesn't take a rocket scientist to figure this one out, folks.

Let's sum things up more broadly. Say your child needs braces, and to make it work out, some permanent teeth must be extracted. You can choose a treatment method that will, in the end, provide an attractive face; a broad, full smile; and will require only one surgery to remove four teeth (the second molars). Or you can select the traditional treatment method and, essentially, gamble on the final result, hoping your child isn't left with a less-attractive face, a smaller smile, and two surgeries for the two different sets of teeth removed (four bicuspids then four wisdom teeth). Remember, it's a free country. The choice is up to you.

(To yours truly, it's an easy choice.)

More formally, the clarion advantages of the second molar extraction technique for children and teenagers (where indicated) can be summarized as follows. Keep in mind this is only when extractions of those teeth—for certain types of malocclusion—are truly indicated.

Advantages of the Second Molar Extraction Technique

- Preserves the arch width of the front teeth at the corners of the mouth so that the lips remain full, supported by both a greater number of teeth at the corners as well as by center front teeth that aren't constricted inward by traditional metal braces.

- Very easy on the patient and incredibly safe—that is to say, it represents a low surgical risk since the second molars are always easier to get at; requires a much shorter and easier recovery time.

- Removes only four teeth, the bicuspids are saved (preserving the fullness of the lips and face), and the third molars are put to good use.

- Frees up key space. (In the traditional treatment plan for braces, removing the bicuspids at the corners of the mouth does absolutely nothing to help dis-impact the third molars way in the back. They're still just as jammed in their respective sockets. Thus, once the orthodontic treatment is complete and the braces come off, the patient often must then be referred to an oral surgeon for the frequently difficult extraction of four additional teeth [the third molars]. Extracting bicuspids creates space to de-crowd teeth in the front of the mouth; it does not create any extra room in the back, where the wisdom teeth already are fighting a losing battle. Second molar extraction, however, does.)

- Is much simpler—and safer—than the extraction of third molars, a common necessity for young adults that can be painful, expensive, and unduly complicated (ask anybody who's had their lower wisdom teeth dug out!).

- Helps solve the underlying problems. (Removing bicuspids from the corners of the dental arches for orthodontic reasons can sometimes compromise the long-term, full-developmental functional integrity of the jaw joints. This can lead to their progressive—and sometimes painful—destruction. Such deterioration is caused by the metal braces and the *orthodontic mechanics* [type of tooth movement those braces represent] that necessarily follow bicuspid extractions as well as the final type of bite [occlusion] the extraction creates. Metal braces are always needed after bicuspids are extracted, but fixed metal braces can't realign lower jaws or change the

(Continued)

dysfunction of surrounding jaw muscles. Only European-style removable oral functional appliances can realign "crooked" lower jaws and refurbish the chewing muscles. All of which is a huge help in making metal braces work better. Therefore, the "European way" results in a more properly fitting bite that nearly guarantees no long-term undue pressure and/or damage to the patient's jaw joints during chewing.)

- Produces a final result that almost always enhances the rehabilitation and ultimate healing of already-damaged jaw joints; preserves and protects those joints that already are in normal health.

- Greatly enhances post-treatment stability (the tendency for orthodontically moved teeth to stay put) because the second molars (the "push-forward experts") are removed and replaced naturally with the third molars (which don't exhibit the same "push-teeth-in-front-of-them-forward" effect).

Remember—and this is extremely important—not every child suffering from jumbled, twisted, or crooked teeth qualifies for second molar extraction (for example, it is usually used only in adolescent patients). But for those who really need it, this orthodontic technique can work wonders.

SIX

The Last Gasp

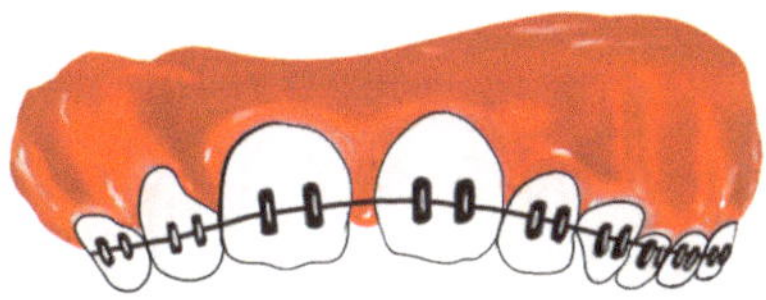

... to sleep: perchance to dream:
ay, there's the rub ...

— *Hamlet*, William Shakespeare (1564-1616),
English playwright and poet

As if all these advanced treatment methods weren't enough, new scientific information has recently emerged—information that will change the world of orthodontics forever. And it concerns, oddly enough, your child's ability to breathe properly during sleep.

When young, growing children are asleep, Mother Nature intends for them to breathe through their noses with their mouths closed. Which might get you thinking, *Well, that's natural. That's the way it always works*. But that *isn't* always the case. And when a child doesn't breathe in the way prescribed by Nature, there can be serious repercussions. It's a very sneaky problem.

Nature designed the human airway systems to work in a specific way. Yes, after strenuous exercise when the body's oxygen demand is at its peak, humans breathe through their mouths—and rather deeply and quickly—to (temporarily) increase airflow to the lungs to meet that demand. But under normal circumstances, Nature wants individuals to breathe through their nasal passages. Have you ever wondered why the inside of the nose is designed the way that it is? It's meant to regulate both the temperature and the humidity of the air we breathe. The inside air passages of our lungs are always moist. Why, then, don't these moist inner linings freeze when we take a breath of -10°F air on a crisp winter day? Answer: The nasal passages condition the cold, below-zero air, allowing us to inhale it safely. Of course, it's more complicated than that, but the design intent of the airways essentially comes down to that critical purpose. Nature generally wants the air we breathe to arrive via our nasal passages—and, most importantly, to do so in proper amounts.

When nasal passages become constricted or even totally blocked, Nature grows increasingly upset, especially when those constrictions occur during sleep. Nature is then forced to strain the chest and throat muscles in order to breathe. Which is bad news!

Recently, scientists have come to understand the significance of this problem and have dubbed it *sleep-disordered breathing*, or SDB. It can lead to major problems, especially in children. It's triggered by things such as a *deviant nasal septum* (crooked or improperly shaped nose bones), large adenoids, and, especially, over-sized tonsils, which restrict airflow through the nasal passages during sleep. Throw in things like allergies—which make the tissues swell up even more—and suddenly the child is in harm's way.

Pediatric or adolescent sleep apnea can result. During this condition, the child stops breathing altogether for several seconds at a time ... followed by a sudden gasp as the body strains for air ... only to stop breathing again a few moments later as the cycle continues.

As you can imagine, not good.

The reason SDB is a serious problem for children is that it often prevents the child from reaching adequate levels of deep, restorative sleep. Those necessary levels belong to what scientists refer to as *stage three sleep*. Similarly, SDB and sleep apnea themselves contain several levels, graded according to their frequency and severity.

(A) 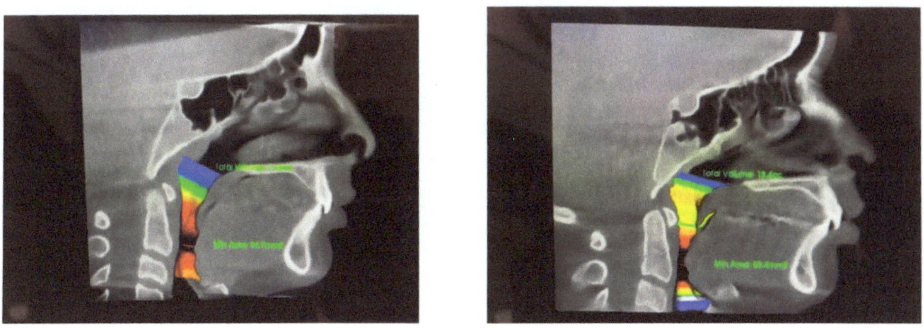 (B)

→ Figures 6-1 (A, B): This pair of images shows a young female patient who received traditional orthodontic treatment at an orthodontic specialist's office in the Midwest. The traditional, metal braces-only type of treatment that she received happened to involve the commonly employed extraction of upper bicuspids, one on each side of the upper dental arch, followed by forcible metal brace retraction of the upper front teeth, moving them back to meet the more retruded lower front teeth. There were no extractions performed on the lower arch, which means the upper arch is as short, front to back, as possible, while the lower arch stretches out as long as possible, front to back, due to all the teeth being present. This particular type of metal braces treatment often results in the lower dental arch—and, subsequently, the entire lower jaw that holds those teeth—being deflected backward too far when the patient bites down. This can prove detrimental to the patient's temporomandibular joints as well as to the upper breathing airway. Figure A is a pre-treatment *cone beam computed tomography* (CBCT), a modern, computerized type of X-ray that is very detailed and, hence, very revealing. This CBCT measures the size of the patient's upper breathing airway (see the dark black section between the red zones, just to the right of that big triangular neck bone). The space measures, at a minimum, 94.7 square millimeters.

Figure B is a post-treatment CBCT of the same patient, five years later. Remember: Only traditional, metal brace-type orthodontic techniques were used, in conjunction with the dual extraction of upper side teeth, one on each side, to allow the metal braces to force the upper front teeth back to couple with the lower front teeth (instead of bringing the entire lower jaw—with its passenger teeth—forward to meet what should have been a non-extracted and, in turn, more-forward upper dental arch).

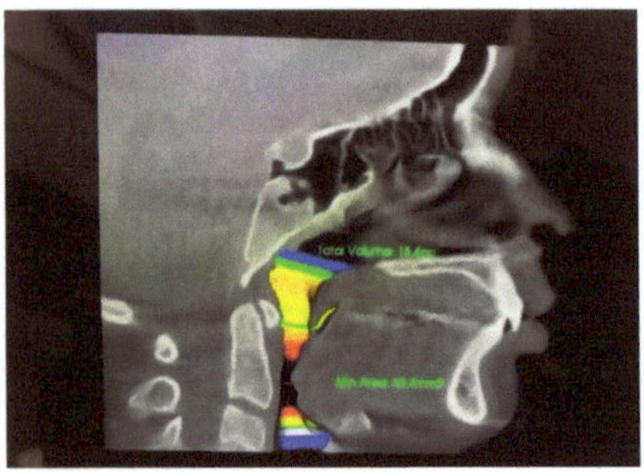

(B)

→ Figure 6-1 (B): Notice how the post-treatment CBCT depicts the upper breathing airway (the now-smaller dark black section between the red zones) after the upper side teeth were extracted and the upper front teeth had been retracted, thus locking the mandible in a more-backward functional position. This image reveals the minimal size of her breathing airway is now only 53.4 square millimeters (i.e., an airway that has been constricted to nearly half the size of the pre-treatment original, which was already slightly less than normal!). Note: These images were taken at full occlusion (full normal bite). What caused this, and how often does it happen?

Special Note: *Sleep medicine experts* (doctors who deal with sleep disordered breathing problems, which, on occasion, can be quite serious) have determined that a minimal cross-sectional area of the upper airway—adjacent to the back base of the tongue—that is less than 100 square millimeters is a major red flag, one that portends trouble! This unfortunate young lady couldn't even meet that minimum prior to her traditional orthodontic treatment, which may well have worsened the discrepancy. Not good!

Some of the conditions that can accompany SDB include the following:

- Circulation and blood pressure irregularities (in severe cases)
- Daytime sleepiness and fatigue
- Diminished excretion of growth hormones (which are produced during stage three sleep)
- Enhancement of ADHD (*attention deficit/ hyperactivity disorder*), if already present
- Jawbone growth deformities and malocclusion (crooked teeth)
- Memory loss
- Poor academic performance
- Prolonged bedwetting (*nocturnal enuresis*)
- Reduced ability to concentrate
- TMJ problems associated with an overly retruded lower jaw that can cause headaches—and even pediatric migraines
- Unusual or increased irritability and other behavioral problems

The term *obstructive sleep apnea*, or OSA, is used to describe the more severe cases.

Why does SDB cause crooked teeth? It's a complicated matter, but, for simplicity's sake, think of it this way. When a child can't get air into his/her lungs in the normal manner (i.e., through the nose) due to some form of perpetual nasal airway and/or *laryngeal* (back of the throat) blockage, the first thing the child will do, unconsciously, is to start breathing through their mouth, especially during sleep. Such a compensation method, subconscious or otherwise, can lead to an overworking of the chest and neck muscles, subjecting them to a steady strain of exertion that also affects the jaw muscles.

As we learned in previous chapters, improper muscle forces on those tender, developing jaws warp their growth such that they can become deformed and even misaligned—top to bottom and/or side to side. This, in turn, means the teeth in those affected jawbones can't help but to come in crooked or misaligned (what we call a malocclusion). Again, the crooked teeth are victims, not perpetrators. Which is why, for these types of malocclusions, you need "fixers" dedicated to both bone and muscle, and not just teeth (such as traditional metal braces). Healthcare providers need to account for any type of SDB problem a child may be experiencing and take appropriate measures to ensure the breathing airways are not restricted to any serious degree. If those airways *are* constricted, they need to take steps to ensure the air passages in the nose, the upper throat, and the windpipe (*trachea*) are of sufficient size to facilitate proper unrestricted airflow during sleep.

Indicators of SDB

- A face noticeably canted to one side or the other (one eye/ear combination higher than the other)
- A highly attached *lingual frenum* (tongue-tie)
- A retruded or weak-looking chin
- A rolled-forward shoulder posture in conjunction with a forward-head posture
- An upper dental arch form that is gothic or arrowhead-shaped in outline (instead of in a gently rounded dental arch form)
- An upper lip that seems too short at a resting, relaxed facial posture to be able to reach the top of the lower lip without straining the lips
- Narrow air passages as seen on a front-to-back head X-ray
- Repeated long-term snoring, wheezing, gasping, or any other breathing-associated noises during sleep
- The type of bite where the front teeth can't touch top to bottom when biting together on the back teeth

The diagnosis of SDB requires examination by a trained healthcare professional who is familiar with the condition. Probably the best place to start is with a dentist trained in the diagnosis and treatment of airway problems. A more formal method of diagnosis involves sleep studies conducted at a hospital or a sleep-specialty clinic (it can turn into a hassle, but, for serious cases, it's well worth the time).

Fortunately, simple and economical home sleep study kits are now available from most healthcare professionals. These are handy ways of obtaining necessary sleep data, at home, in only a few nights. Such tests can establish the diagnosis of SDB with certainty. This paves the way for proper treatment.

(A) 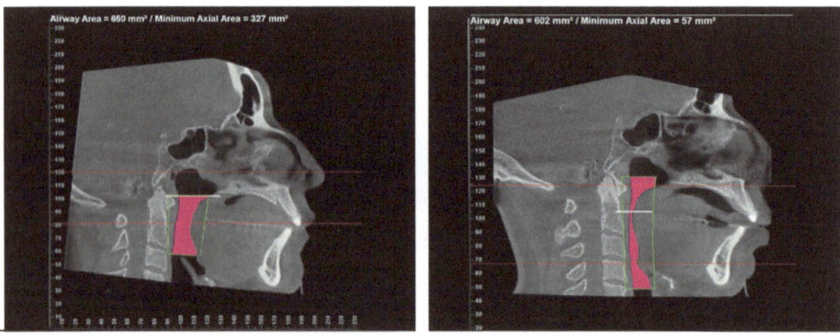

(B)

→ Figures 6-2 (A, B): Here are another pair of CBCT images that show even traditional adult bite guard treatment for TMD is not always free from some of the upper breathing airway complications associated with traditional jaw joint and facial pain treatments. These before and after images depict a 57-year-old male patient who received *TMD splint* (bite guard) treatments. The treatment consisted of the use of a traditional, custom-made removable upper splint that was snapped on to his upper teeth in an effort to drive the lower jaw back and up in its own sockets when the patient bites fully down on the splint. In the past, many specialists believed this type of splint design was a good one—one that would, when the patient bit down upon it, supposedly deflect the entire lower jaw back into its own sockets by preventing the natural fit of the bare, non-splint-protected bite from forcing the jaw joints to seat improperly. They believed the natural bite could somehow traumatize the jaw joints, which, in turn, would cause the pain within them.

So, this traditional bite guard treatment, based on older theories, was supposed to relieve jaw joint pain and other symptoms (those early specialists' ideas were so near, and yet so far!) which led to misconceptions around locking the mandible back during traditional orthodontic treatment (i.e., with metal braces). Of course, now we know better.

In Figure A, the patient is holding his lower jaw in a biting position, one that feels the most comfortable to him for breathing (i.e., a little bit more forward). The problem is, in this biting position, although his back teeth do touch, the biting surfaces of the upper and lower dental arches are quite worn down vertically, top to bottom. This is referred to by dentists as lack of vertical dimension of occlusion. But if the patient bites down any further back, the bite fit and lack of VDO drives his lower jaw backward—and hard. The patient also has been diagnosed with mild sleep apnea; this is a bad combination.

(**Note**: The average person bites their teeth together about 1,500 to 2,000 times per day. Often, that's because that is simply how many times per day most people swallow [i.e., every time they swallow, they generally clench their back teeth together]. And that number isn't counting the chewing, grinding, or clenching of teeth during intense periods of stress, nor the gritting of teeth during sleep!)

Because of chronic facial pains, sore jaws muscles, painful jaw sockets, and chronic, recurrent headaches, this patient sought help at a major Midwestern university. As stated above, they fashioned him an old-style, removable intra-oral TMD splint in an effort to relieve his symptoms. But guess what: It only made them worse! The patient remarked that, while wearing the splint during the day, his lower jaw pains were much more intense; and, while wearing it at night, he couldn't properly breathe and had to strain to get air through his nose. As a result, he was forced to open his mouth to breathe, thereby disturbing his sleep.

The patient could only bear wearing the splint for about a week before the discomfort got so intense that he had to remove it completely. Frustrated with their own failed attempts, the doctors at that same university are now saying he needs upper and lower jawbone surgery to bring the jaws forward to help open up the upper-back part of the breathing airway.

Such a procedure would entail them first cutting loose the entire upper jawbone, teeth and all, and wiring it together in a more-forward position. The aim of this is to accommodate the surgically advanced lower jaw and its passenger teeth, which would, in turn, help move the base of the tongue more forward (it's currently residing in a trapped and obstructive position), thus opening up additional space between it and the upper airway.

There is only one problem with this approach—and it's a big one! The only way to surgically advance the mandible is to first cut it in half. The front half is moved forward and wired-in to heal, dragging the attached base of the tongue with it and thus opening up the airway. But the back half of the lower jaw, on each side, must be seated firmly in the jaw sockets before it can be wired in place; some surgeons take rather robust measures to accomplish this. And, of course, this forceful placement does absolutely nothing to help a patient's damaged jaw sockets, which are already jammed back too hard at full bite.

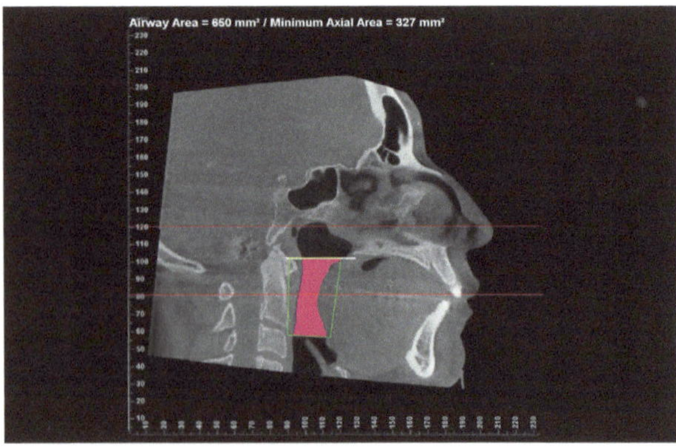

(A)

→ Figure 6-2 (A): As mentioned previously, this image shows the manner in which the patient likes to relax and "naturally" posture his lower jaw for comfort. The upper airway (in pink) measures, at a minimum, a robust 327 square millimeters. Nature likes that!

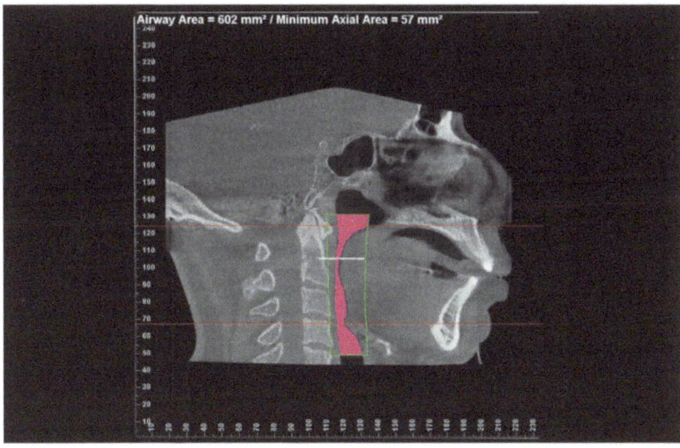

(B)

→ Figure 6-2 (B): This image shows the upper airway while the patient is biting down onto that university-made removable intra-oral bite guard. Again, recall that the patient could only stand to wear this splint for about a week before the increased pain and breathing difficulties caused him to stop! The upper airway in this "post-treatment" CBCT image measures, at a minimum, a mere 57 square millimeters: a reduction of 82%! Also notice the accentuated curl of the lower lip's profile (*mentonian groove*), a sure sign that the lower jaw is back too far.

(**Additional Note**: As of this writing, the patient is *still* awaiting the university-recommended complete upper and lower jawbone surgery, which his insurance company refuses to pay for! Hopefully, he will be able to find a clinician with the skills and experience necessary in order to get his jaws and their sockets working properly—and done so non-surgically. I know; it's hard to believe, isn't it?)

I bet you can't guess what treatment for SDB entails! Our medical colleagues generally go the *adenoidectomy* and/or *tonsillectomy* route. For us dental experts, however, treatment usually involves proper orthodontics: producing lateral upper dental arch expansion (sideways)—and, if need be, maybe even forward realignment of the lower jaw itself—to allow more room for the upper windpipe to open up. (Moving the lower jaw forward creates a new, more-forward bite that automatically drags the base of the tongue with it. This corrects its original rearward operating/resting position, where all that *lingual musculature* was pressing against—and thus constricting—the upper airway.)

The above treatment techniques come directly out of the modern functional orthodontic playbook. Moving the lower jaw forward (when needed) not only helps with facial beauty, but also helps improve constricted airways for proper breathing. All of this relieves strained or jammed temporomandibular joints, which, because of their misalignment, may already be causing the affected child to suffer from headaches—and, yes, even migraines.

Help for these suffering children is finally at hand.

Hallelujah, indeed!

SEVEN

FJO, TMJ, and the Big Headache

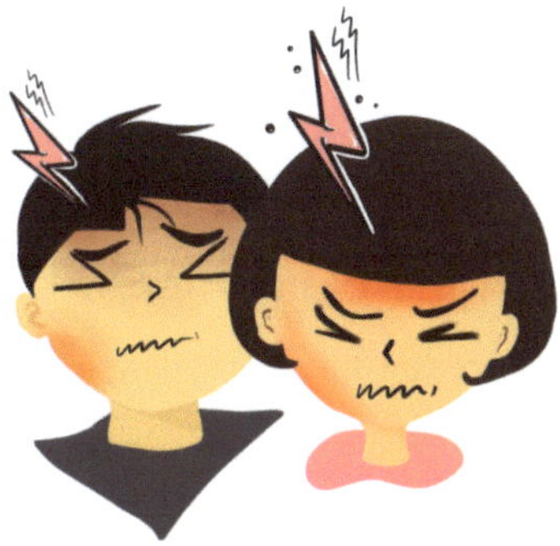

Truth has no special time of its own. Its hour is now, always, and indeed then most truly when it seems most unsuitable to actual circumstances.

— Albert Schweitzer (1875–1965),
Franco-German physician and
African missionary

A note for readers: You may think this chapter will be a big headache since it's a bit long and a bit technical, but I promise all of it is important material that will help you protect your child and give them the very best in dental healthcare. Moreover, the concepts below aren't as difficult to understand as you might think; they only seem that way at first. After you digest the information, you'll see that it's all just a matter of common sense, and that it represents one of the most important medical/dental breakthroughs concerning the long-term health of your child and/or yourself!

I know what you're thinking: "All right, so there are a few new ways of doing braces nowadays. Great. But why am I spending all this time reading this confusing book? What's the fuss really all about?"

While it's true that not every case treated with conventional-style metal orthodontic braces ends up producing a caved-in face, a flattened smile, or a retruded profile (even when four bicuspids are extracted in the old manner), it's simply not worth the risk. Some cases do turn out well; others, however, don't. Far too many, as a matter of fact. What if your child is one of them?

The "orthodontic look" on young teenage faces is still quite prevalent today, though it shouldn't have to exist at all. But there's a still-deeper issue to contend with, something far more important—and far more sinister—at work. It's a relatively recent discovery, albeit one that was made over several decades in piecemeal fashion. But its arrival on the dental scene has been cataclysmic. Its significance will change the way we look at the traditional orthodontic (metal brace) technique as well as the functional jaw orthopedic (FJO—or, European-style removable appliance) treatment methods forever. It's a problem that's surprisingly ubiquitous, appearing in a sizeable percentage of the general population of orthodontic patients (both children and adults alike), and it's serious enough to adversely alter a patient's overall quality of life. It is a problem that has an enormous economic and social impact, causing the kind of suffering that can interfere, change, and even ruin lives. It is pernicious. It is relentless. It is one of the great evils ever to befall the health of humankind. It has stood for centuries unchallenged, hovering over humanity like a dark-hooded specter of merciless suffering. The mere mention of its name strikes fear into the hearts of its hapless victims.

What is this vile menace, you ask? It is the sickening, excruciatingly painful form of headache known as the *migraine*.

But have no fear: The dental community has miraculously stumbled on what now truly appears to be a real—and permanent!—migraine cure. It is a remedy that has shocked all of us in healthcare, lending new meaning to the debate over modern methods of performing orthodontics (a debate that is sometimes referred to by its slang term "Jaw Wars"). This cure is also amazingly easy to explain to laypeople; paradoxically, it's surprisingly hard to explain to educated dental folk. While bedeviled with details, it is, in essence, an incredibly simple concept, one with a success rate so high that even its own discoverers couldn't at first believe it. But, in the final analysis, it is a cure that makes perfect sense, thanks to the "high-tech" knowledge recently discovered by our colleagues in neurology. Can you guess what this miracle cure is?

The human temporomandibular joint.

It's a big name for such a little piece of anatomy. It is a jaw joint socket residing back by the ear, where the horseshoe-shaped lower jaw attaches to either side of the base of the skull. Its name derives from the two major bony components that comprise the jaw joint. The human skull is a fusion of many bones; the area above and to the front of your ear is often informally referred to as the "temple" due to a bone—about the size of a common coffee cup saucer—located there. In scientific lingo, that bone is called the *os temporale* (in Latin, the word *temporal* means "time"; the bone's name, then, refers to the fact that the side of your head is where gray hairs first start to appear).

The *os temporale* not only protects the temporal lobe of the brain but also contains the ear hole (known as the *external auditory meatus*) and the ball-and-socket-type hinge of the jaw joint, positioned just ahead of the ear. It's composed of a smooth, rounded, bony socket, one that's big enough to easily fit the fleshy part of your thumb. The socket itself is shaped like an upside-down shot glass, with a thicker, rounded front edge. (Its medical name is *glenoid fossa*, or just *fossa*, which means "bony depression" or "socket.")

This bony socket makes up one piece of the jaw joint, the stationary half that is part of the skull. The mandible—or the two end sections of it, anyway—make up the other part of the jaw joint, the movable half. As mentioned in prior chapters, the lower mandible is a horseshoe-shaped lower jawbone with two rounded balls of bone at either end. These rounded ends form the *ball* piece of the ball-and-socket jaw joint combo and are referred to as the *mandibular condyles* (or just *condyles*). They fit nicely into the bony fossae on either side of the skull. Hence the compound name temporomandibular ("temporo" + "mandibular") joint—or, TMJ for short.

There also is a little disc of cartilaginous fibrous tissue inside each jaw joint. Called the *articular disc* (*articular* means "internal joint"), this tissue rides between the condyle and its partner fossa and is only about the size of a nickel. The disc is thick and rounded at the edges, while thin in the middle. It acts as a shock-absorbing biological cushion between the top part of the condyle—which goes into the socket, traveling back and forth during opening, closing, and chewing—and the inner bony surface of the fossa.

Since both the mandibular condyle and the edges of the socket are rounded, the surface arrangement is mechanically unstable from an engineering standpoint. The cushioning effect of the articular disc works in a fashion similar to cartilage cushioning discs in your spine.

No matter the joint, Nature doesn't like bare bone rubbing against bare bone. When bone-on-bone friction occurs—if the workload is great enough and goes on long enough—it wears down the opposing surfaces of those bones (and sometimes even makes them noisy). Then the bones and tissues around them become inflamed and sore (*arthritis*). All of which explains the universal presence of shock-absorbing cartilage—or a similarly tough gristle-like tissue—in areas of skeletal bony joints, where the opposing bones grind against each other with a forceful load during function.

The TMJ's articular disc sits forward slightly over the front of the condyle's rounded head (like a Frenchman's beret cocked forward). It's situated this way so as to always remain between the lower jaw's ball-shaped condyle and the inside rim of its bony fossa (socket). As the lower jaw opens and closes, the down and forward movement of the condyle causes it to slide back and forth over the front edge of the socket, a natural part of the process. When the mouth is opened wide, the condyle is positioned a bit out past the socket's rounded front rim. That's okay, a completely normal position at full opening. The condyle does the exact opposite during closing, moving back into the depths of its own socket in an up-and-back fashion. This back-and-forth movement of the condyles during opening, closing, and chewing is called *translation*. What's important to note is that when the lower jaw opens and closes, the condyles don't "rotate" in their respective sockets; rather, they "translate" in and out, backward and forward. The articular disc moves, too, always protecting the opposing bony surfaces.

Or, at least, that is what's *supposed* to happen.

While the articular disc fits snugly against the top of the condylar head, it is *not* directly fused to it. Additionally, the disc is slippery and wiggles around somewhat as the condyle translates during lower jaw movement. This means the articular disc can sometimes be torn loose or otherwise damaged—or even fully dislocated—by certain types of forceful or repeated trauma. It then becomes what is referred to as the *slipped disc* of a bad joint. Such slippage in joints—whether it occurs in the jaw or in the spine—has great neurologic ramifications. The nearby nerves get involved, sometimes being abused due to the displaced disc. When slipped discs occur in the spine, patients usually suffer backaches. When slipped discs occur in the jaw joints, something entirely different occurs.

Which leads to an oddity worth noting: The actual size of the fossa in humans (and even in some animals, like horses) is always just a tad bigger than it needs to be in order to cradle its respective mandibular condyle. It's like a shoe that's three sizes too big for the foot inside of it. What does this mean? Plenty! How is the condyle supposed to fit in its fossa when that socket is a bit too big for it? How does it know just where to position itself when it fits in there so loosely? The answer: Nature has a way.

The condyle of the lower jaw is programmed and designed to stay fairly tight against the inner forward edge of the socket, in both rest and function. Tiny ligaments inside the fossa tether the joint disc in place. Thus, it can ride along with the condylar head quite a distance, down and forward, during a wide mouth opening.

The condyle's normal starting point in the socket is where it and its companion disc reside when the mouth is fully closed. The special ligaments within the jaw joint are specifically designed—and strategically attached—to prevent any excessive up-and-back, jamming-type condylar movements, which would drive the ball deeper into the upper cavity of its oversized fossa. Shoving the condyles too far up and back is bad news, which is why Nature tries to prevent it with those little, limiting internal joint ligaments. Repeated jamming of the joints can damage and tear these protective tendons. Then the jaw sockets can get overly jammed. That's bad news!

All in all, the TMJ mechanism is a gristly conglomeration of cartilage, ligaments, and connective tissue that's extremely tough. It has to be. It takes enormous abuse (look at what prize fighters go through!). However, the accumulated everyday strain sometimes can become too much for the joint, typically in sneaky ways, over a long period of time. When it finally gets bad enough—especially if it receives extra abuse like a good hard blow to the chin—the patient's internal joint structures consequently break down, sometimes rather quickly (or even instantly as in the case of sudden trauma). That's when the true trouble starts—and in more ways than one.

When the jaw sockets break down internally due to chronic, long-term damage caused by the wrong type of biting and hard-chewing forces, all kinds of joint pain and other troubles result. When this happens, patients are said to have *Temporomandibular Disorder* (or TMD). Sometimes, the associated pains can be great.

This degenerative jaw joint condition is, to dentists, sort of like Mark Twain's comments about the weather: Everybody talks about it, everybody has an opinion on it, everybody thinks they know something special regarding it, but few people ever completely understand it—or try to do anything about it. The same was true for years in the world of TMD. At least until now!

More than 50 years ago, back when I was just a young student in dental school, if I'd wanted to write a term paper on TMD, I would've had a tough time. You see, believe it or not, there were no books on it back then. Oh, sure, there were chapters (or parts of chapters) about the condition found in books on *oral pathology* (the various diseases of the mouth and jaws), but there were no real definitive sources, no "bible," so to speak. There was nothing to consult that would tell you exactly what was happening to the TMJ when it broke down—nor, more importantly, was there any information on how to fix it (non-surgically) when it did happen. Back then, dentists couldn't even agree on what to name it.

TMD, while painful, is actually a very simple condition that requires many complicated factors working in concert to form. When it occurs, it manifests itself in a variety of complicated—and often agonizing—ways, which made it difficult for dentists of the past to solve. But, out of the chaos, patterns of signs and symptoms gradually emerged. Some of them held big surprises.

The concept of TMD as a *pathological* (or disease) entity was first officially put forth in the '30s by an *otolaryngologist* (ear, nose, and throat specialist) named Dr. J. B. Costen. But TMD didn't really arrive in the collective dental consciousness until the '60s. Back in those days, due to the complexity of the problem, doctors really didn't understand what TMD was, nor could they agree on what type of treatments (and there were many) would temporarily alleviate it—or finally cure it. All they knew was that something went wrong deep inside the sockets of the jaw joints, resulting in varying degrees of pain in the face and the jaws. It also triggered a physiological breakdown of the joint's internal components (again, to varying degrees and in various stages).

Because of this slow, steady process of internal breakdown within the socket, the patients would suffer tremendous discomfort, including head, neck, facial, ear, and jaw pain. Beyond that, it was a scientific crapshoot as to what TMD actually was and what was really going on with these patients. In those early days, one doctor's opinion was about as good as another's. It seemed like every time you kicked over a log, out hopped a self-proclaimed TMD expert. Most believed something in the bite interfered with the mandible's closing path to "the fully locking bite," thereby transmitting some sort of improper and/or excessive shock forces to the jaw joint's internal components, bringing about their eventual breakdown.

Other culprits were blamed as well, with psychological stress being one of the leading contenders. Everybody had their favorite "trick" method for treating what they believed was TMD. They took dental drills and ground off high spots from the biting surfaces of the back teeth to smooth out the bite. They used pills. They shot medicines directly into the affected joint. They tried biofeedback, tranquilizers, physical therapy, and jaw exercises as well as cold, heat, and various other forms of stress-relieving techniques. They fiddled with the patient's diet, tried prescribing vitamin and mineral supplements, and, in the most desperate situations, even limited the patients' diets to only soft foods (as if that would truly solve anything). And, of course, surgeons got involved by cutting the joint open and figuratively saying, "Oh, look, the disc is torn loose from its normal location and displaced way down and forward in the socket. It has sort of slipped out of place. And look, there are also lots of little torn ligaments all over. It's a black-and-blue, shredded-up mess! To fix it, we'll take out the disc (maybe) and sew everything back together again. Everything will be fine."

They did. It wasn't.

Oh, sure, some of the patients saw improvements, sometimes going pain free for six months to a year after the reparative surgery.

A few of the lucky ones got permanently healed. But, for other patients, a terrible thing happened. The jaw and facial pains reappeared, persisted, and generally, in the long run, got even worse!

Understandably, TMD surgery didn't exactly earn itself the best reputation at first. Those fortunate patients who recovered—whether surgery or another of the various early TMD treatment techniques were used—probably did so by accident. Nonetheless, the success of any particular treatment convinced the attending doctors that their favorite TMD treatment trick was the real answer. More likely, they were all at least partially right.

Just about any treatment technique—as long as it made some sort of scientific sense—would probably help at least some of the patients, at least some of the time. For a while, anyway. But nobody had a technique that worked every time on every case. It was a nightmare for patients and doctors alike. Failure and frustration reigned supreme. Soon only the bravest of doctors would even attempt to tackle TMD, what was becoming known as a diagnostic and therapeutic "black hole." There seemed no real way out.

The constant, day-in/day-out jamming of the loose condyle can lead to the disc itself tearing free and squeezing forward, off the front edge of the condylar head. This produces an arrangement of fully closed and occluded lower back teeth interlocked against the upper back teeth at full jaw closure but with a resultant *internal derangement* of the jaw joint's internal articular disc (with the condyle seated too deep, up and back in the confines of the socket). Put simply, that makes for a joint that's dislocated and, as you can imagine, any dislocated joint is never a good thing. When the dislocation occurs internally and the joint is continually overworked, that's even worse.

Mother Nature will respond in the only way she can: with pain!

When a patient has a severely dislocated and inflamed jaw socket and they bite down together, hard, all the way, they are in effect repeatedly dislocating their own joints, causing themselves undue pain and perpetuating the joint damage.

TMD is classified as a *syndrome*. A syndrome is a group of signs and symptoms that seem to go together. Over the years, dentists have gone so far as to host entire conferences just on how to categorize what they thought were all the many kinds of TMD. If a patient's jaw hurt *this* way, it was called one kind of TMD; if it hurt *that* way, it was dubbed another. Complicated classification charts were devised, and picking just the right name for the related symptoms became a mark of the "TMD elite."

After all, according to all those concocted diagrams and charts, there were a dozen or so different kinds of TMD conditions to choose from. And since these doctors couldn't go to the biomedical library and look up the real answers in a textbook, everybody treated the problem *empirically* (medical lingo for "by the seat of their pants"). Which is why, in the old days, they had whole committees of dental and medical specialists who worked with seriously affected TMD patients. Hosted at clinics associated with big university medical centers, the committee usually would consist of a dentist, an orthodontist (maybe), a *gnathologist* (a dental occlusion or bite-fit specialist), a nutritionist, an oral surgeon, and, of course, a clinical psychologist (or even an M.D. psychiatrist, because "half of those TMD patients are crazy. It really is, most often, just a *psychosomatic* problem."). Bunk!

Because of the confusion and clinical wheel spinning, the murky world of TMD treatments became a medical/dental "no-man's-land," where only the boldest clinicians dared to tread. It also resulted in a form of empirical "TMD turf"—i.e., a way of viewing the problem that often was a product of emotion rather than science. In other words, various TMD schools of thought sprang up around the country, each championed by various high-profile dental and/or medical leaders. Each school was often theoretical in nature, founded more on considered opinion than on scientific and *pathophysiological* fact. Since they were so strongly entwined with the proponents' particular pet outlook, such viewpoints regularly were defended in a jealous and emotionally charged fashion, each camp blind to any criticisms or rival forms of thought.

As a consequence, ego supplanted altruism in the TMD treatment world. Doctors worked *against* each other rather than *with* one another. It was as if a clinician's personal worth as a healer—and even as a person—was irrevocably intertwined with their ability to defend a particular position on the TMD issue. Meanwhile, the truth—and the patients—continued to suffer, shoved aside by stubborn-minded TMD doctors of various stripes, all in an effort to make clinical reality fit their particular preconceived idea (rather than vice versa).

In this regard, highly trained professionals are, in some respects, no different than common people. What happens when you take a stubborn, narrow-minded person who has a propensity to be a "stick-in-the-mud" and give them a fancy, highly technical education? You get a highly educated, stubborn, narrow-minded person who has a propensity to be a stick-in-the-mud! The world is full of them—or at least it seems so. Which leads to the point that being smart has absolutely nothing at all to do with being right. But not to worry. There are also heroes present. In fact, most individuals in this business are in the latter category, but there are enough in the former to occasionally cause all the rest of the professionals a lot of trouble.

It wasn't just one doctor, or one school of thought, or one scientific event, that brought about the discovery of modern, effective approaches to correctly understanding and treating TMD. The knowledge just sort of evolved over a 30-year period, though of course there were key players and events. For the sake of brevity, however, we will discuss this great and complex scientific evolutionary process collectively, in overly condensed symbolism. I will describe it as if the discovery took place all at once and was accomplished by only one (mythological) dental doctor. The important thing is that you grasp the main concept. We've come a long way together so far in this little book; it's now more important than ever that you stick with me on this.

The first real candle in the darkness was lit (symbolically, if you will) when one intrepid TMD clinician stood up at some national seminar and said, in effect, "Hey, everybody. Guess what? There really aren't a dozen different kinds of TMD—there's only one! At least only one that we dentists are chiefly concerned with: the condyle/disc dislocation type of TMD."

He continued: "Classic, garden-variety TMD is a product of a bad-fitting bite in the patient's jaws, the sort that causes the lower jaw's mandibular condyles to jam too hard up and back into their own sockets at the powerful end of full bite. That process gradually—and sometimes not so gradually—destroys the joint's protective cushioning disc and supportive ligaments inside the socket. This turns *really* bad when, at the worst of times, a repeated crushing force by the hard bony head of the condyle is employed, causing serious damage to a vulnerable group of little arteries and nerves that just happen to reside in the upper back parts of the jaw socket. It is these bruised, crushed, and damaged nerves (and their accompanying blood vessels) that are—in a drawn-out, round-about way—the true source of the patient's pain."

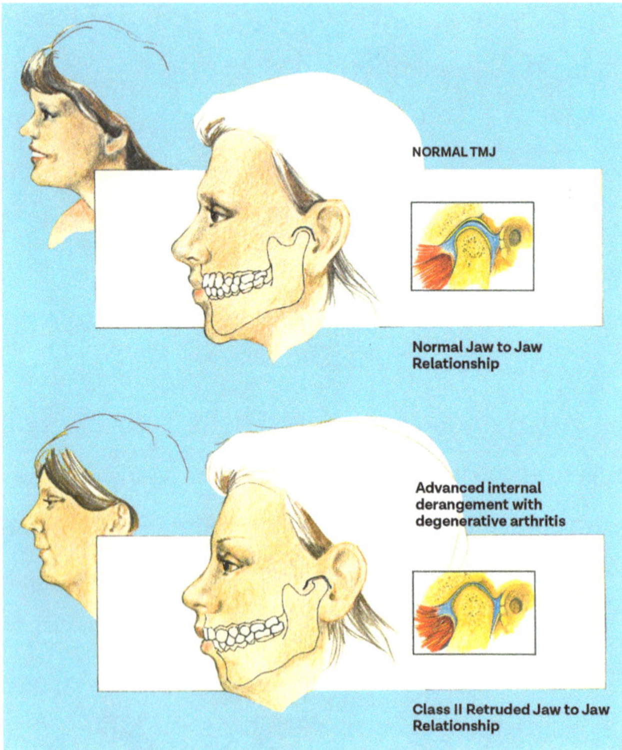

7-1

→ Figure 7-1: The upper image of this illustration depicts the contours of the mandible's condyle as well as the proportional clearance between it and the bony socket that cradles it. In the lower image, you see a patient with TMD; note how tight and jammed the condyle is within its own socket, to the point where the arthritic (joint damaging) changes that can occur actually deform the living bone of the joint. This can result in chronic, recurrent TMJ pain, facial discomfort, headaches, and the entire family of migraines. Also notice how, in the bottom image, the patient's lower lip and chin profile are a little further back, in both a Dental and Skeletal Class II alignment. Compare this to the picture above it: a proper Class I upper-jaw-to-lower-jaw alignment, featuring a proper fit of the upper and lower teeth. You can also make out the disparity in shape between the normal bony condyle and deformed, abnormal, arthritic condyle. Years of dysfunctional abuse (jamming) by a backward-deflecting, and trapping, bite would be necessary to deform the bone this much. Dentists call this type of bony degeneration *osteoarthritis.* The facial pains and headaches this condition cause can really make patients suffer! In the meantime, the body tries to fight it off and adapt. Sometimes, it does a pretty good job of this; sometimes, it doesn't. And that's when the pains begin.

He went on, adding, "Yes, there are many manifestations of this problem. In fact, if you want to get really fussy, no two TMD patients are exactly alike. It's similar to female pregnancies. No two of them are the same, either. But, if you look at 1,000 pregnancies, you'll be able to find a general pattern. And even though it's somewhat variable in nature, it's still remarkably predictable."

Then, this mythological doctor dramatically concluded: "It's that way for TMD patients, too. They exhibit an extensive, yet fairly common (and somewhat variable), pattern of signs and symptoms. The most common of which are chronic, recurrent headaches. Even these, the headaches themselves, can vary between patients, exhibiting all types of intensity, frequency, quality, description, and location. They can range from a common, mild, tension-type headache (occurring only once a month), all the way to the pounding, prostrating, and extremely painful migraine-type headaches, with all their accompanying bizarre neurological symptoms. But it is the chronic, recurrent (primary) headache, in the absence of any other general medical cause, that is the chief calling card of TMD."

It was a bold statement. As you might guess, the dental community figuratively gave themselves headaches from laughing so hard when they first heard this. The healthcare profession as a whole had a tough time accepting this new and radical paradigm, which directly established the TMD-migraine connection. For many, it was simply too big of a pill to swallow. (The only thing that's actually funny in all this is that the patients themselves never have much difficulty understanding the concept. They're just focused on getting well!)

But progress didn't stop there. An even bigger, and more stunning, revelation followed on the heels of these initial TMD headache cause-and-effect discoveries. Not only did these intrepid pioneering clinicians tell the world what TMD actually was; they also promptly proceeded to share the solution!

What they proposed came as an even bigger shock. They said a bad bite that perpetually jammed the lower jaw too far back against its sockets—damaging (or bruising, if you will) all those varied small nerves and blood vessels—caused the repeating headaches. Therefore, creating a new bite—a slightly more forward-fitting bite for the lower jaw, just enough to decompress the mandibular condyles and keep them operating safely—will stop the chronic compression of nerves in the upper back part of the socket, which is the real culprit for TMD's headache and facial-pain problems.

Once the bad bite has been corrected, the bruised nerves and torn ligaments in the joint gradually will "scar over" and eventually heal. Consequently, the headaches will not only soon cease, but never return! It was a sensational cause-and-effect theory that ran contrary to centuries of thinking. This, as you can imagine, didn't go over well at first. Few could (or would) believe it. Most rejected it. Arguments ensued.

Critics scoffed and said, in effect, "This 'condyle-jamming-up-and-back-too-far-during-full-force-biting business' isn't what TMD really is. And moving the fit of the bite and the whole lower jaw permanently forward several millimeters—then forcing it to stay there and effectively work in that new position—won't really cure chronic TMD-based headaches, jaw pains, or TMJ damage and degeneration, let alone migraines. Even if it somehow would help, it can't be done. You can't realign an entire lower jaw to fit more forward and keep it chewing in that realigned, more-advanced position. The body won't allow it. The jaw muscles and the internal joint structures won't take it. The whole idea flies in the face of the time-honored concept of the patient's life-long, habitual bite positioning. In sum, this isn't what TMD is, the treatment technique won't work, and, more than anything, it simply can't be done."

They were wrong.

(A) 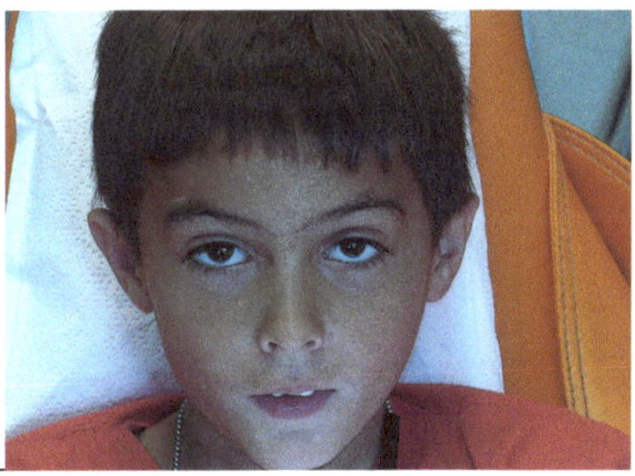

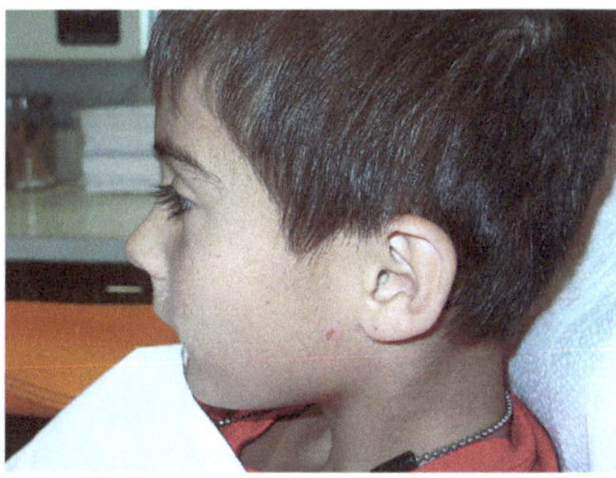 (B)

→ Figures 7-2 (A, B): This kind and gentle 10-year-old boy was diagnosed with both a Dental and Skeletal Class II malocclusion (lower teeth *and* lower jaw further back than their properly positioned counterparts) as well as a Condylar Class II (lower jaw jammed too far back into its sockets at full bite).

(Continued)

Both of his upper and lower dentitions were gothic in outline, with a noticeable point to the front (like a tall, thin church window) instead of the proper rounded, more Roman-arch outline. This reflects an upper jawbone shape problem as well as a front-to-back, upper-jaw-to-lower-jaw alignment issue. As a result of this untoward combination, the patient also suffered from sore jaw sockets, tender facial and jaw muscles, and both *T-type* and nascent migraine-like headaches—and at only 10 years old! Observe, in the pre-treatment profile, his recessed lower jaw.

(C)
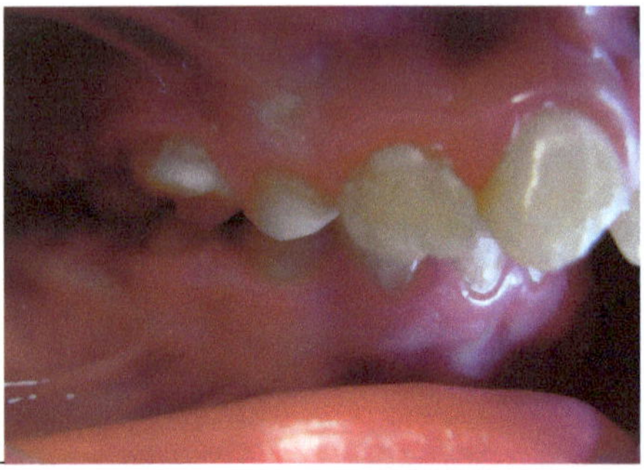

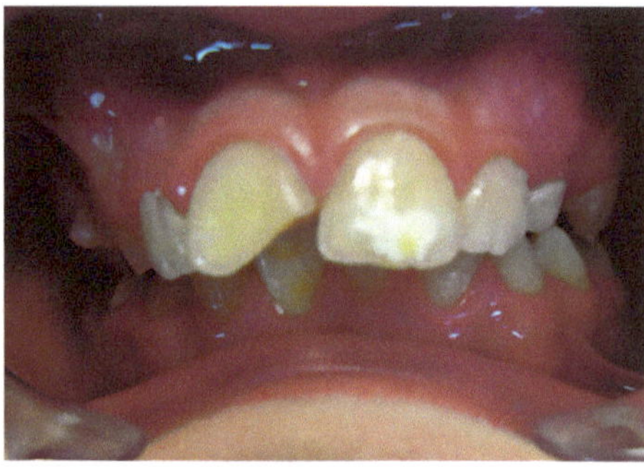
(D)

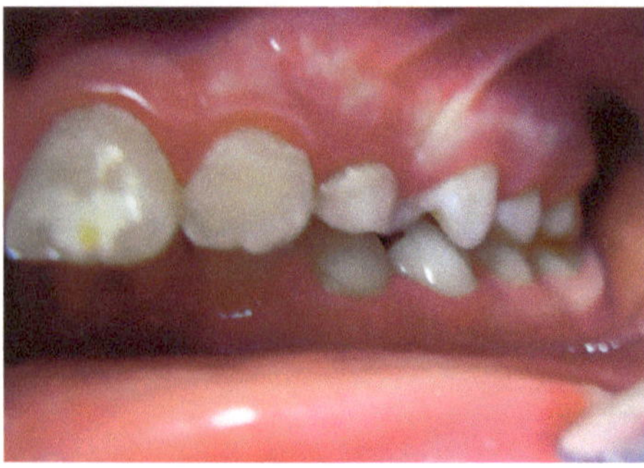
(E)

→ Figures 7-2 (C - E): Frontal and right-and-left quartering views of the pre-treatment malocclusion. (Notice the hockey stick "erosion" on the patient's upper-right front tooth—after all, he's a Minnesota kid!)

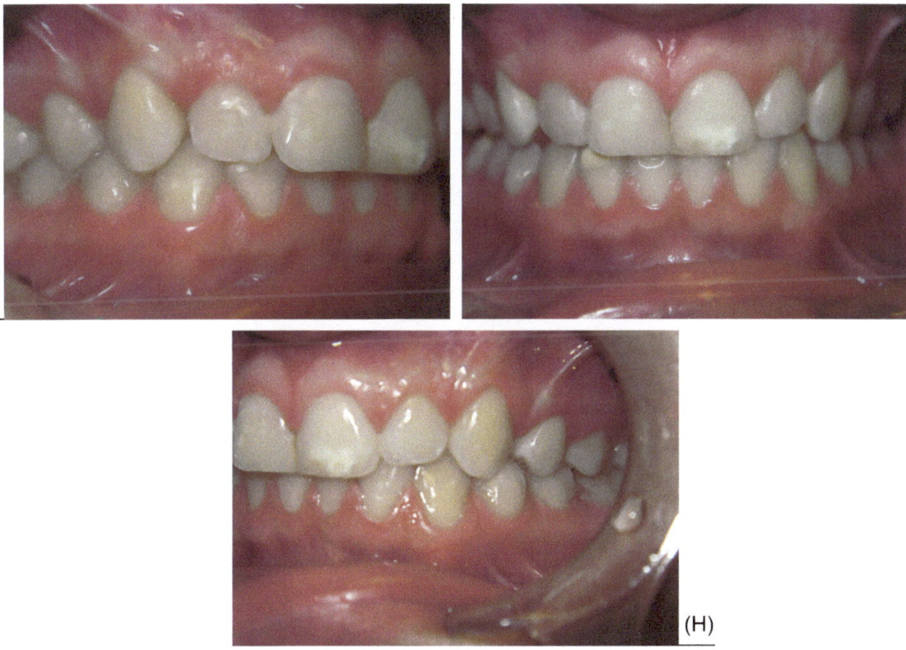

(F) (G) (H)

→ Figures 7-2 (F - H): The patient's post-treatment corrected occlusion, which is a result of conventional functional jaw orthopedic and orthodontic methods, using exclusively removable appliance techniques (i.e., no metal braces were needed!). The TMD headache and jaw pains were completely eliminated—early within the treatment, in fact—and were never to return.

(**Note**: That broken upper-front tooth was fixed with modern restorative dental procedures.)

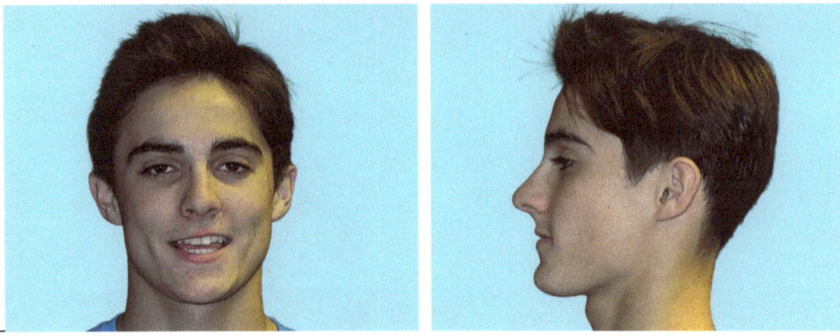

(I) (J)

→ Figures 7-2 (I, J): Final post-treatment facial views, both frontal and profile. Compare Figure 7-2 (J) with Figure 7-2 (B). And, best of all, no headaches!

The proponents of the new approach were right, pointing to the work of their European colleagues, who had demonstrated that realigning displaced lower jaws *can* be achieved through the use of their removable functional orthodontic appliances. It all seemed too incredible to believe. (Even *I* couldn't believe it 40 years ago when I first heard of the new approach.)

As a TMD-treatment concept, it was revolutionary, to say the least. Many experienced experts still have a tough time choking it down. But, due to advances in technology, it has all been proven true, time and again. Which means the world of TMD (and the treatments used to combat chronic, recurrent migraine) will never be the same, neither will the discipline of orthodontics for children.

Things are certainly changing in this business. Now it's just a matter of who can keep up. Science is like the proverbial "time and tide." It waits for no man. Some of its biggest revelations can catch us off guard—that can't be helped—but it's our duty to learn and to adapt.

The recently discovered (and scientifically proven) concept of the TMD-migraine connection has arrived—with or without anybody's permission—and is now here to stay.

And that's news to celebrate!

EIGHT

Why the Big Headache?

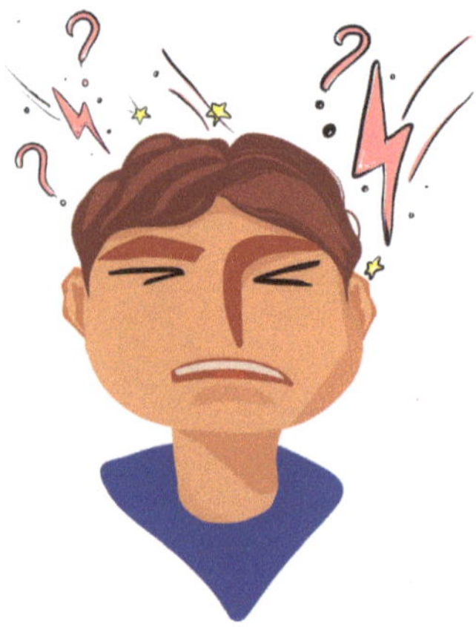

It is the cause, it is the cause, my soul,—
Let me not name it to you, you chaste stars!—
It is the cause.

– *Othello*, William Shakespeare (1564-1616),
English playwright and poet

For those of you who suffer from chronic, recurrent headaches, or have a child who suffers from them, this chapter will prove incredibly important to you. It is the heart and soul of this entire book. The content may seem difficult because of its technical nature, but that's why I taught you all the preceding material, so you can understand what's to come. Again, the majority of this will be overly simplified for the sake of clarity, though it'll still reap enormous dividends in helping you understand why you or your child suffer from the various types of TMD-induced headaches.

Let's begin.

Numerous conditions besides TMD syndrome can cause chronic, recurrent headaches. Most of them are easily diagnosed by general medical protocols (for example, if a patient has a brain tumor, diabetes, *lupus erythematosus*, or some other systemic disease that leads to headaches, the underlying cause can usually be deciphered easily enough). Of course, we've all experienced a common headache before, whether it was because of a bad cold, a bout with the flu, or a sinus infection. This is not the kind of headache we're talking about. The headaches we're concerned with here, as described in the previous chapter, are the kind related to crushed, bruised, and damaged bundles of nerves/blood vessels in the upper rear portion of the jaw socket. These headaches are chronic, recurrent ones—of any quality, variety, intensity, or location—that cannot be associated with any other general medical cause. They often are accompanied by various forms of neckache and/or upper shoulder aches. They are termed "primary" headaches.

Hyperalgesia is a neurological pain-processing term that describes an exaggerated or heightened perception of a painful stimulus. Strike your thumb with a hammer, for example, and the next day your thumb will continue to throb, demonstrating a hypersensitivity to stimuli. Same with a sunburn. Get fried at the beach, and the next day your sunburned skin will be hyperalgesic. Chemical processes that take place inside the pain-transmission nerves—processes that are perfectly natural—account for this phenomenon. Hyperalgesia usually lasts until the damaged tissue fully heals. Then the exaggerated pain response fades away.

Heterotopic pain is another sophisticated neurological term for an important pain-processing phenomenon. It is known commonly as a "referred pain pattern." Headaches often fall under this category. During this phenomenon, pain is mistakenly *perceived* (felt) by the patient as coming from a different location in the body than its actual source. For instance, people suffering from a heart attack often sense not only a crushing-type pain in their chest during the event, but they also often perceive a severe (referred) pain radiating down the inside of their left arm. There is absolutely nothing wrong with their left arm, but that's where their brain feels the impulse. A slipped disc in the lower back often produces a similar effect, this time with referred pain radiating down the leg (*sciatica*). Once again, there's nothing actually wrong with the patient's leg, but that's where the pain feels like it's coming from nonetheless.

Heterotopic pain, then, is a sneaky pain-processing neurological trick Mother Nature likes to play on us, one that can sometimes fool doctors and patients alike. It usually occurs when pain nerves have been *sensitized* by overuse, a process that makes them hyperalgesic (as previously described). That isn't to say referred pain isn't *real* pain. It is. Even though the patient swears they are feeling discomfort in a place where it's not actually coming from, the pain isn't made up. All of which can drive patients and their treating doctors nuts when trying to figure out what's really going on!

In the case of TMD, the jaw sockets undergo a type of long-term, compression-type nerve damage to an *arborization* (branching) of a group of very important pain nerves and their accompanying blood vessels. This artery complex, by some sort of anatomical bad luck, happens to pass right through the inside upper portion of the socket's bony dome, which cradles the condyles of the movable lower jaw to the side of the skull. It represents a true from of a *neuroanatomical* design flaw—one of the few in the entire human body.

For the unlucky nerves and blood vessels that must squeeze through that part of the socket, it's the equivalent of being stuck "between a rock and a hard place." The constant unprotected pounding this area (called a *neurovascular bundle*) has to endure when the jaw joints aren't working right sets up a scenario in the back of the socket that neurologists have come to define as a *chronic compression nerve damage model*—not a good thing at all. Normally this problem can't happen unless there's some form of abnormal internal ligament damage and disc derangement (slippage forward, or out of place in its own socket). Although these nerves in the jaw socket are small, continually irritating and harming them can result in significant consequences. How tiny are the nerves on the surface of your eye? Get a grain of sand in there and see how *those* little nerves respond!

These repeated jaw/nerve pain impulses from the poorly working jaw joints may at first be so sneaky and so subtle that the patient might not even feel them or be aware of their presence (neurologists call this phenomenon *subclinical input*). But the brain, at deeper subconscious levels, sure knows it's happening. Except for the conscious part, the brain (in its deepest subconscious) never sleeps. It's always aware of what's going on throughout the body. As such, when these repeated pain signals from the bruised nerves accumulate to a certain level (called *threshold*), the brain reacts in special neurological ways. Given enough time—and enough buildup—this process "fries" the neurological circuitry of some of those pain transmission nerves as well as some of the brain's other related pain transmission circuitry.

It's as if the nerves themselves become neurologically "sunburned" (or, hyperalgesic). Neurologists call this overall process *sensitization*, caused by numerous complicated chemical reactions that occur in individual nerve cells (known as *neurons*). As a result, pain generated through TMD (which may only really be a two on a scale of one to ten) has the potential to feel much worse than it is (say, a five or a six).

For TMD patients, there are three main sources of headache pain: from the jaw muscles; from the internal structures of the jaw joint itself; and, most importantly, from the blood vessels of the inner parts of the brain. For reasons yet unknown, there exists—in the massive and complex pain nerve system of the human head—a complicated, built-in neurological reflex that is *automatic* (not under any sort of voluntary control by the patient). When activated, this reflex—along with other less extensive but interconnected neuronal pain-processing reflexes—can "act up," triggering side effects that can really do a number on a patient with TMD damage (including simple headaches and even migraines).

Pain anywhere in the body—whether from trauma, infection, etc.—usually implies some form of tissue damage, which Mother Nature doesn't like and makes you subsequently pay for in the form of pain. And if you keep it up, such that a repeated pain-generating situation leads to pain-nerve sensitization, she's going to see to it that you *really* pay—which means increased, exaggerated, and prolonged discomfort that spreads out from the original area of damage (hyperalgesia and heterotopic pain).

Bad news!

All major muscles in the body (except for the muscles that govern facial expression) pull from one bone to another across a joint. Muscles never push; they only *contract* (or pull). When a particular joint gets damaged, the related muscles often tighten up (similar to the way in which the muscles in your lower leg stiffen when you sprain your ankle). This, too, is a neurological reflex, beyond a person's voluntary control. When muscles stiffen up in this way, they are said to have increased electrical-type muscle tone or *tonicity* (or to be *hypertonic*). (This is an extension of a physiological principle called Hilton's Law, after an old-time physician who first discovered it over a century ago.) The worse the internal joint damage, the more the muscles reflexively tighten in an effort to stabilize, protect, and heal the injured joint. It's as if the muscles are saying to the injured joint, "I am going to hold you still so you can more easily recover." The body tries hard to take care of itself—sometimes in strange, yet ultimately clever, ways.

The same principle comes into play when the temporomandibular jaw joint is involved. Enough severe joint socket damage can initiate various levels of reflexive jaw muscle tension, leading to muscle pain. As they stiffen, those jaw muscles tend to shorten, which in turn holds the lower jaw progressively more closed and retracted during non-chewing intervals (referred to as *mandibular rest*). This, in turn, keeps the pressure of the condyle tighter on the now-already bruised and slightly swollen nerve complex within the back portion of the socket, thereby generating even more pain impulses. Due to Hilton's Law, these impulses then automatically call for more muscle tightening and spasms, pushing the condyle microscopically deeper still into its own socket (resulting in still more compression and pain) in a vicious cycle that feeds on itself. It's no wonder patients with TMD syndrome frequently can have sore jaws, sore facial muscles, and accompanying headaches (the headache being an example of the previously described phenomenon of referred or heterotopic pain).

At first, the pain-feeling centers in the brain attempt to hide (or somewhat ignore) all of this. The body has natural, built-in pain-fighting centers that continually work to filter out or tone down all varieties of aches and pains. But these pain filters can't do everything. When the brain reaches a point where it can no longer repress the accumulated signals from the sore jaw joint and its tensed-up muscles, it often erupts in a referred pain pattern in the form of a headache (of any quality, intensity, location, or duration). All regular headaches then—and even the far more painful migraines—are a kind of heterotopic pain.

Yet it isn't all doom and gloom; there *is* some good news. Nature, in her infinite wisdom, is well prepared to deal with long-term pain assaults that stem from various parts of the body. The brain's pain filters are constantly at work. Often, a patient may not be aware that TMD degeneration and chronic compression nerve damage is even occurring. In addition, the patient may not consciously perceive a problem until the sheer cumulative low-grade pain signals overwhelm the filters in the brain. At that point, conscious pain perception begins, usually in the form of jaw pains and/or generalized headaches. The natural pain-blocking mechanisms in the nervous system can then get even more overwhelmed, and the formerly mild (tension-type) headaches now escalate into the full-blown whoppers known as migraines. The symptoms of TMD-migraine syndrome are about to reach their zenith.

When a certain neurological threshold in the brain's nervous system is reached, the blood vessels of the brain (not *all* of them, mind you) reflexively tighten down or temporarily *constrict*. This act reduces blood flow in certain key areas of the brain, causing it to behave funny until the blood vessel tightening (or *vasoconstriction*) relents.

Depending on the severity and specific location of this temporary, reflex-generated constriction, certain areas of the brain's circulatory system can get "starved for blood." *Focal neurological phenomena* follow suit, a fancy name for transitory symptoms that some patients experience right before or during a severe migraine attack.

These symptoms can include:

- Certain types of minor hallucinations
- Dizziness, pallor, weakness, and/or fatigue of the muscles of the head, neck, or—in extreme cases—even other parts of the body
- Nausea
- Seeing jagged, wavy, sparkling lines
- Temporary blind spots or partial loss of vision
- Tingling in the fingertips and ringing in the ears
- Tiny floating spots of light flowing through a patient's field of vision
- Unusual sensitivity to light, sound, or smells
- Vomiting

After a brief period of vasoconstriction, or localized diminished blood flow, the brain says, in effect, "That's enough of this baloney. I want more blood, and I want it now!" With that, the affected blood vessels, reflexively over-constricting at the time of the headache, are ordered (by a special neurologic directive from other more powerful centers of the brain) to *dilate* (or widen). This process restores normal blood flow in the affected areas; however, it also has negative effects. The neural signal from those commanding brain centers is so powerful, and so sudden, that the poor overtightened, over-constricted blood vessels rapidly course correct, stretching themselves wide open and over-dilating. This always hurts. And it's not an isolated, sharp pain, either; it's more of a profuse, sickening, deep ache. To make matters worse, the pain signals travel right back around to the brain, through the chemically jacked-up (sensitized) pain nerves of the head and their related neurological junction boxes (which themselves have been sensitized due to processing an abundance of signals from the damaged jaw joints).

The cycling of these amplified pain signals further feeds the migraine headache attack process, which then calls for more prolonged and painful reflexive dilation of those same blood vessels in the brain, widening and stretching them even harder, making them more painful while feeding yet more signals back through the same pain nerve loop, over and over, again and again.

This is why patients suffering a severe migraine sometimes can feel their every heartbeat pounding through the painfully dilated blood vessels of their head. Such migraine pains can be profusely referred anywhere throughout the brain, often perceived as a throbbing, pounding ache around or behind the eyes. The head, the jaws, the neck, the inner ears—all are afflicted. Sometimes even a patient's back teeth hurt. The patient swiftly grows tired, nauseated, and crabby—i.e., just plain sick. Meanwhile, constant TMD pain processing and related neurological reflexes continue to cycle out of control in a sensitized head-pain-nerve system. It's a mighty misery, indeed. The old-time doctors called all this a "nerve storm."

The location, severity, and duration of the repeated headaches—from simple, mild (tension-type) headaches that involve the temples and other muscles of the jaws, all the way to the pounding, prostrating, vomiting migraines that involve pain from dilated, inflamed blood vessels—are an indicator of how much previous TMD damage exists inside the jaw sockets, how long it has been there, the level of host resistance, the type of joint damage involved, the amount of reactive neurological and chemical sensitization that has taken place, and many other factors that can neurologically feed the TMD-headache reflex. (There are a vast number of factors, especially in women. Female sex hormones can really fire this up. It's not fair, but that's just the way it is.)

The TMD-initiated headache pain neurological reflex eventually will exhaust itself (and the patient) and usually subsides (although it is common for a true migraine attack to last up to 72 hours). Then, like a smoldering volcano, it all starts again: building and building until the next eruption. It may take weeks or months, or—in more advanced cases—it may take only a few days to reach its threshold once more, when another painful headache outbreak occurs.

Special headache medicines can break the pain cycle and bring temporary relief, but they are no real permanent cure. Other physical modalities sometimes can help, too, but they only mask or hide the syndrome, unable to permanently eliminate it at its source. For some lucky patients, Nature *might*—as in, *possibly*—eliminate the TMD-generated migraine reflex process on its own, over a period of years. But this seldom happens in females, and even when it does, as previously stated, it can take years or even decades. No one knows precisely how long, or why this occasionally occurs.

For most patients, the pattern of repeated headaches (of both types), accompanying jaw aches, and various other pains continues on for decades, with the headaches returning again and again—day after day, week after week, year after year—often growing in strength, frequency, and intensity. Medicines can only do so much and only for so long. They attack the effects (pain) but not the cause (TMD). And every medicine comes with its own collection of side effects—which, with repeated long-term use, often can become a serious secondary problem in its own right!

One more thing: People with TMD hold their heads forward by about 10 degrees. Never mind why; they just do. Usually, they don't even know they're doing it (it, too, is a subconscious reflex). Now, the adult head weighs about 10 pounds in smaller females and 12 to 14 pounds in larger males. It's perched precariously on top of the spinal column, girdled by a ring of neck muscles that keep it erect. With prolonged instances of poor head posture—as TMD patients often exhibit—the neck muscles become overworked, overtired, and, subsequently, become stiff and sore.

And guess what? They feed their sensitized, pain-carrying nerves right up to the same pain-sensing relay centers in the brain, through the same pathways and junction boxes and neurological circuitry that the head and the jaws use. This is one of the important reasons why certain TMD patients (especially females) can universally suffer from chronic, recurrent neckaches of one degree or another along with their repeated headaches.

The Importance of a Proper Jaw-to-Jaw Relationship

1. Most Important - Upper-Jaw-to-Lower Jaw Relationship

2. Secondary Importance - Upper-Teeth-to-Lower-Teeth Occlusal Relationship

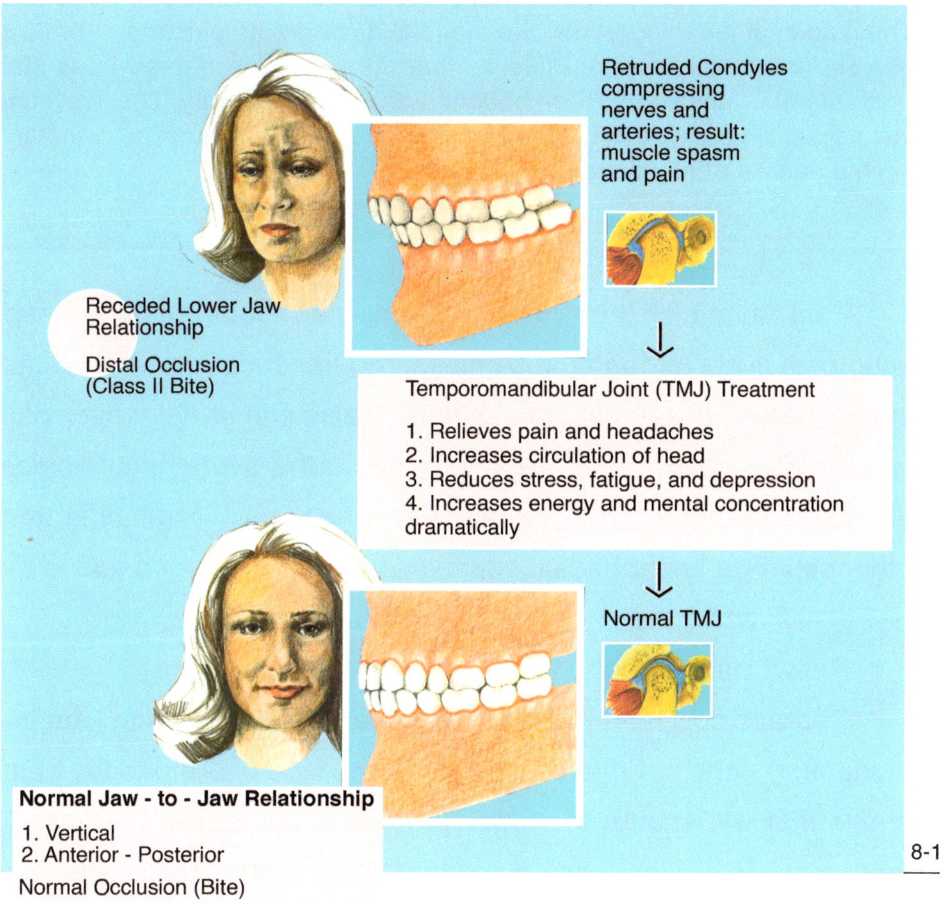

→ Figure 8-1: Illustration showing the significance of the jaw-to-jaw relationship (dictated by the fit of a person's bite) and the resultant TMJ conditions that such relationships might affect. In the upper image, the woman

shown has a Class II malocclusion; notice how all the lower teeth and the lower jaw are pushed back from their upper counterparts (observe the step between the lower and upper back teeth). Also notice how tight the spaces are between the condyle of the lower jaw and its socket (just in front of the earhole). This tightness is the result of damage from the Class II bite (or its equivalent), and it can cause nerve damage to the nerves passing through the back of the socket, which then leads to facial pains, TMJ pains, headaches, and even migraines. In the lower image, the woman has a correct Class I (normal) bite; notice the lack of backward step between the upper and lower back teeth. The fit of the teeth at full bite is correct, and there also is more spacing between the rear of the condyle and its socket. Thus, no joint jamming at full bite, no joint damage, no pinched or bruised nerves, and no headaches! (Remember: The average person bites their teeth together anywhere from 1,500 to 2,000 times per day. The teeth and jaw socket anatomy, then, really need to fit properly in order to withstand such a degree of functional stress.)

Pain stemming from stiff neck muscles feeds into the headache-pain cycle through the same shared transmission boxes, making the headaches even more intense. It also can transfer neck pain to the head, *anywhere* in the head, due to the overall neurological effects of TMD. Experiencing additional neck pain originating from other separate, independent sources in the neck can also add to the issue, worsening the entire thing.

Phew! Had enough?

Perhaps now it makes sense why dentists "in the know" are tremendously concerned about delivering the kind of orthodontic treatments that will ensure the lower jaw winds up positioned properly forward while straightening a crooked set of teeth. Getting the jaws "right," way back at the jaw socket level, helps cure any existing internally deranged TMD-pain-headache cycles that might already be present (or hiding just below the surface). It also makes critical progress, in a child or an adolescent, toward preventing such a cycle from ever becoming established in the first place, ensuring that the finished bite helps secure the lower jaw's condyles properly within their sockets.

If a patient suffers from recurring headaches induced by a steadily degenerating set of temporomandibular joints, rebuilding the bite—by moving the whole lower jaw (and hence its condyles) slightly more forward into a permanent chewing/biting position—will eliminate the repeated jamming-type biting pressure on those small nerves at the rear of the socket. This prevents the villain of chronic, compressive nerve damage from constantly recurring in the jaw joints, miraculously allowing the reactive chemical changes occurring inside the joints' nerve cells—which play a part in the transmission of both intensified and referred pain—to chemically revert back to normal, to the way they were before the jaw sockets' nerve damage sensitized them in the first place.

Thus, the chance of a repeated, reflexive over-constriction of the jaw muscles (Hilton's Law) is eliminated. Neurologically, the complicated, pain-generated reflexes in the brain's blood vessels see a reduction in gain and intensity, which then helps eradicate the constrictive blood vessel spasms and corresponding over-dilation in those same vessels. Finally, in almost all cases, the intense referred pain of a migraine attack (felt throughout other parts of the head, especially behind or across the eyes) is quickly diminished and eventually disappears altogether. What a deal!

Many of the various steps (and there are quite a few) in this complicated and exotic cascade of serial neurological events have been carefully documented, piece by piece, by different research centers throughout the world. The only problem is that headache pain researchers and neurologists aren't TMD-oriented dentists; as a result, they don't quite understand the condition of TMD, nor how a damaged set of jaw joints can provide the repeated, degenerative deep-pain source for the related head (and jaw) pain nervous system, which chemically sensitizes the pain-processing pathways and can thereby initiate the "neurological groundwork" for the entire complicated migraine event. These researchers know that chronic compression nerve damage, acting as a deep-pain source somewhere in the head's pain-nerve system, is capable of causing this repeated migraine-headache process, but, as of yet, they don't fully realize that the condition known as TMD is the culprit. They shouldn't feel bad, however. Most dentists don't realize it yet either. Only a few.

But those few will change the TMD/pain/headache world forever. Many are pushing harder than ever to spread this new and controversial knowledge throughout the dental profession by means of books, continuing education symposiums, lectures, seminars, and technical articles in professional journals. (Some of those dentists even talk about it as if they invented it!) This knowledge has the power to benefit the work-a-day dental clinician by making his/her orthodontic and related TMD treatments better. It is knowledge meant to help the suffering patients because, not only will it help clinicians deliver better orthodontic care, but it will also help both children and adults become true winners in the never-ending battle against chronic, recurrent headaches. Like all new, revolutionary knowledge, however, it goes against the grain of traditional beliefs and, thus, arguments ensue. Undoubtedly, it will take a while for these ideas to completely filter down through the extended rank and file of healthcare professionals. And it won't be easy. Massive egos are involved, as you can imagine, and those practitioners who endeavor to propagate this new insight will face enormous obstacles in their path. Despite the fierce resistance from some of their colleagues, in no way are they about to give up. Good thing, huh?

To sum it up as simply as possible: Due to modern technology, we now know for sure that stopping perpetual jaw joint damage—caused by a bad bite that jams the lower jaw too far back in its own sockets—also halts the perpetual headaches, even migraines, that inevitably arise. *That's* the only proven way to cure migraines.

Where are the leaders who deal in this? Although they're not on every street corner, you can find them if you spend but a little time searching. You might even be surprised where you find them. Their numbers, thankfully, are increasing each and every day.

NINE

So, What Does All This Mean (Choice-wise) to Me?

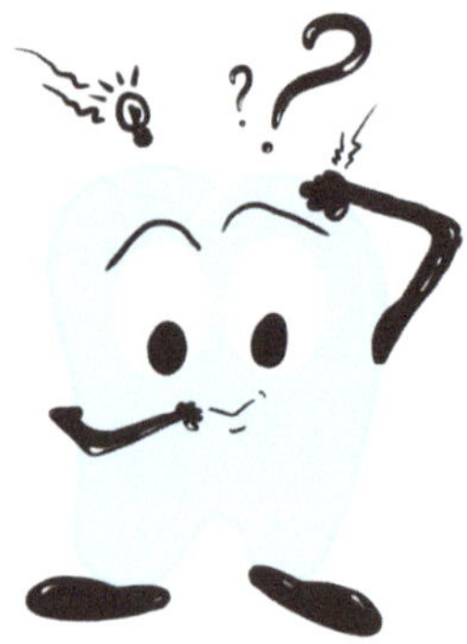

The humblest citizen of the land, when clad in the armor of a righteous cause, is stronger than all the hosts of error.

— William Jennings Bryan (1860–1925),
U.S. orator and politician

For about half of you with children who are in need of braces, this book is meaningless.

Strange to read, perhaps, but honest: The reason these concepts won't apply is because studies show 50% to 60% of children with malocclusions that require orthodontic care have perfectly normal temporomandibular joints. Which means any type of competent orthodontic treatment will usually suffice, including traditional metal braces used to move the crooked teeth. Damaging your child's jaw joints further through improper or incomplete treatments need not concern you. Of course, you may have some apprehensions if the proposed treatment plan involves the extraction of four permanent bicuspids in the traditional way. You may want to seriously think that one over. It may be the right choice for certain cases, but, in most circumstances, there are now other, better options from which to choose. Often, though not always, bicuspid extraction can be saddled with a number of long-term problems, so it is in your best interest to discover what new methods are available for your child.

(You should also be concerned if your child's lower jaw is underdeveloped and biting way back [skeletal Class II], giving the chin and lower face a recessed look as well as contorting the smile with a "buck tooth" appearance. Many times bad bites such as these are *not* a matter of upper front teeth sticking out too far, but rather a matter of the whole lower jaw being undersized and trapped by the fit of the child's upper and lower teeth, which constantly forces them to bite back too far.)

But for the other half of you who seek orthodontic care for your child, this book is *very* important, as numerous studies from around the world show that, on average, about 40% (or more) of all children who require major orthodontic care already suffer from enough TMD damage to be detectable by the examining clinicians, even when those investigators are using only the most primitive and basic of diagnostic procedures. This poses a serious problem. Let's examine why.

One thing you must understand is traditional orthodontic procedures—techniques that involve treatment with only metal braces and wires, used in conjunction with the extraction of bicuspids to gain space in the dental arches and align/straighten the remaining teeth—very often produce an end result that, at best, maintains the same pre-treatment upper-to-lower jaw biting relationship in the jaw joints; or, at worst, causes the relationship to become even more strained and deteriorated because the bite is cinched back even further by the braces and wires as they close up the gaps left behind at the bicuspid extraction sites.

Either way, these traditional, metal-brace orthodontic techniques seldom ever result in the patient's lower jaw coming forward in the final bite; they only appear to do so. Yet for the child who is already suffering from overt jaw joint damage—or who has a hidden kind of damage smoldering below the surface, just waiting to be set off (what TMD experts refer to as *posterior displacement of the condyle at full occlusion*)—the traditional orthodontic treatment scenarios described above are most often flat-out unacceptable.

The reason they're improper for a child with beginning TMD-type problems in their tender, growing jaw sockets is because the treatment will either leave the child's strained, damaged, structurally compromised temporomandibular joints as is, or will cause them to become even more structurally compressed. Furthermore, such treatments will usually not correct the TMD damage already present. The long-term condition of mandibular condyles being driven too hard and too far back into their sockets by the existing bite—even after traditional metal braces have been used to straighten the teeth cosmetically—has an enormous chance, sooner or later, of manifesting in the form of TMD, which then often flares up in the guise of chronic, recurrent, tension-type headaches (or even the more sinister migraines).

Sometimes the joint damage is already so great that the child experiences jaw clicking, jaw pains, and repeated headaches of various sorts, frequencies, and intensities—all before orthodontic treatment has even begun. Sometimes the joints are so crooked from the start that the poor child suffers from a nasty headache condition known as a *pediatric migraine* (studies show about 4%–6% of all children in the U.S. suffer from them).

The Critical 3mm Joint Space

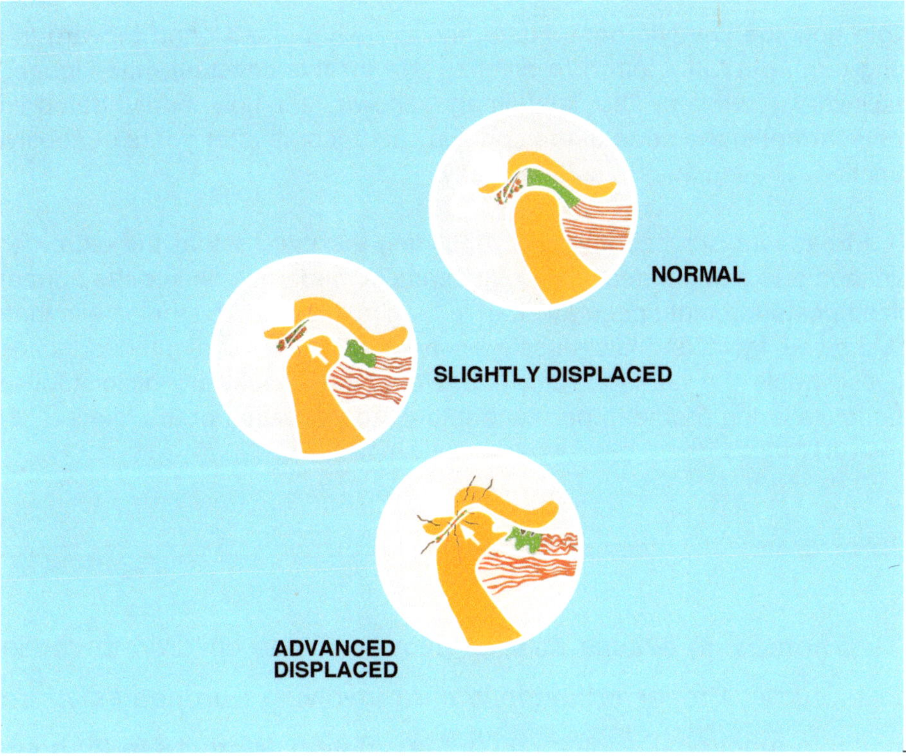

9-1

→ Figure 9-1: Shown here are three schematic drawings representing a TMJ viewed from the right side (outside looking in). In all three, the small white circle represents the ear canal. In the upper right image, the arrow is pointing to the space in the back of the joint at its normal proportional size. The green object represents the tough but flexible disc that acts as a protective shock absorber to the opposing bone surfaces of the socket and the upper condyle. The tiny red and green circles represent the nerves and arteries forced to squeeze their way through the space. The red, string-like objects depict the muscles attached to the bone of the condyle of the lower jawbone, helping it operate properly.

In the middle picture, we see how, at full bite of a malocclusion, the mandible is starting to be driven back too far into the socket. This repeated overclosure and jamming causes damage to the internal joint ligaments. It also squeezes the protective disc forward, out of place, so that the disc's shock absorbing capabilities are lost (Nature doesn't like that). This, in turn, allows for the constant "bruising" of the nerves squeezing through the space. (Nature *really* doesn't like that.)

Note how the condyle bone is starting to reshape and bend forward in a long-term, but futile, effort to compensate for this constant, bite-induced, backward jamming. The final image shows just how badly deformed (osteoarthritis) the head of the condyle can become after years of abusive function. These patients suffer greatly.

The treatment process involves rebuilding the bite so that the extremely pinched and bludgeoned back joint space is made to look like the normal-sized posterior joint space as seen in the first picture. This helps eliminate TMJ pains, facial and jaw muscle discomfort, and, most of all, headaches. It also heals the damaged sockets. Permanent backward dislocation of the joints is the problem; permanent forward relocation of the joints is the answer!

There is no excuse now for allowing these children to continue to suffer. Proper orthodontic care involving European-style removable functional appliances is the solution. Worn 18 to 20 hours per day, these appliances unlock the backward-driving bad bite and gradually—over a period of months—grow the mandible slightly more forward and down (by as little as only several millimeters) to a new permanent bite, one that doesn't pressurize those torn-up and damaged jaw joints, thus eliminating the pediatric migraines, every time. You can take that to the bank!

So, if you play the odds, at least four out of ten of you are up against it. The orthodontic care you select will have a serious impact on your child's ultimate internal jaw joint condition and whether or not that condition deteriorates (or has already deteriorated) to the point of causing chronic, recurrent headaches. It's unfortunate, and it isn't fair, but that's just the way it is. The good news is we can now solve such problems. Knowledge really is power!

What all this means is you should ask your dental clinician what the status of your child's temporomandibular joints are prior to beginning orthodontic treatment. Don't be fooled by a lack of clicking, pains, or headaches; trouble could be quietly brewing below the surface. If the clinician can show you a specific TMJ *radiograph* (X-ray) of your child's jaw joints and explain what these images show, fine. If your child has a retruded chin or buck teeth, with upper front teeth appearing to stick out too far, ask the clinician how the proposed treatment plan will affect your child's facial profile and the lip support around the corners of the mouth—especially if dental extractions of any kind are planned. Also inquire whether such types of treatment could possibly be detrimental to the jaw joints themselves. It's perfectly in your right to ask such questions. It's *your* child.

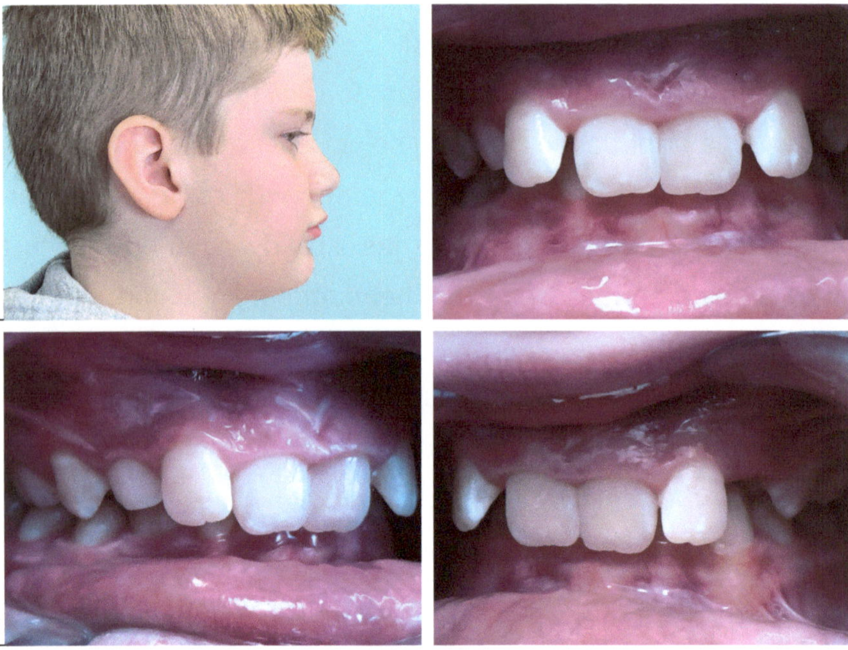

(A) (B) (C) (D)

→ Figures 9-2 (A - D): This 11-year-old boy suffered from terrible, vomit-inducing migraines every other day for nearly two years. His jaw sockets were the victims of a severely backward-deflecting malocclusion. He experienced sore jaw and facial muscles, and his TMJs were so damaged that X-rays showed the bones within them were starting to become arthritic, slowly dissolve, and change shape (a condition known as *regressive remodeling*). By the time these photographs were taken, his condition had deteriorated to such a severe level that he was suffering from extreme migraines on a day-to-day basis.

A simple perusal of the pre-treatment images (Figures 9-2 [A-D]) should instantly make obvious what was occurring. Notice how the lower lip exhibits a profound forward curl (referred to as a deep mentonian groove), which is a sure sign that the bite isn't right. Additionally, the back teeth are also not yet high enough out of their sockets (lack of vertical dimension of occlusion). As a result, the entire lower jaw gets deflected backward into its own sockets during full bite—and way too hard, at that. Notice how in Figures 9-2 (B-D) the lower teeth can hardly be seen behind the uppers. In the sideview pre-treatment images (C and D), the upper lateral incisors *aren't* flared out too far, but are actually in the correct position: angled forward the way they're supposed to be. It's actually the two middle frontal teeth that are improperly angled, positioned too far inward. Upon closing down at full bite, this inward angulation deflects and traps the lower dentition—and the entire mandible itself—way too far back, a condition referred to as a Class II, Division 2, deep overbite (lack of VDO). These types of malocclusions can often prove very harmful.

(E) 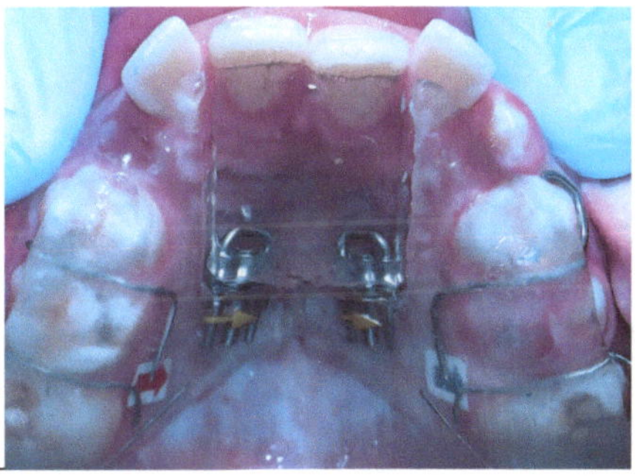

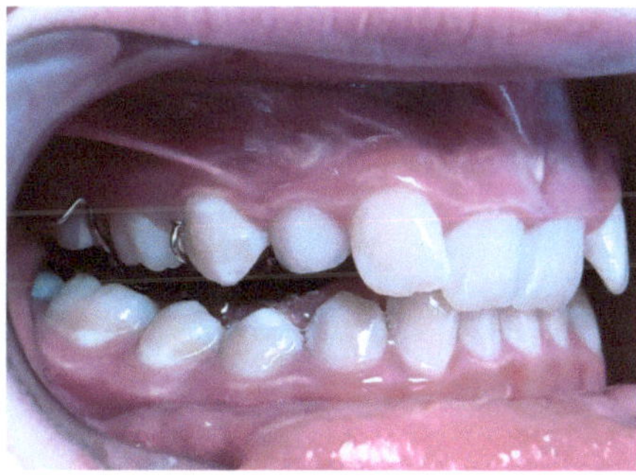 (F)

→ Figures 9-2 (E, F): Treatment began with an effort to correct this exceedingly improper angulation, working to push the two offending upper front teeth back to where they belong. The bite guard portions of this upper appliance (a removable active plate called a *maxillary Sagittal II*, worn on the roof of the mouth) provide both a degree of bite-opening and bite-blocking effect. Hence, it also provides a modicum of TMJ protection, which very often results in some form of headache pain relief! The 11-year-old patient wears this appliance 24/7, eats on it, and removes it only for cleaning, brushing, and expansion screw activation. He turns the little activating screws himself, at home, twice per week, which gradually and gently expands the active parts of the appliance in quarter-millimeter increments. Thus, the offending upper two front teeth are correctly angulated in several months.

(Continued)

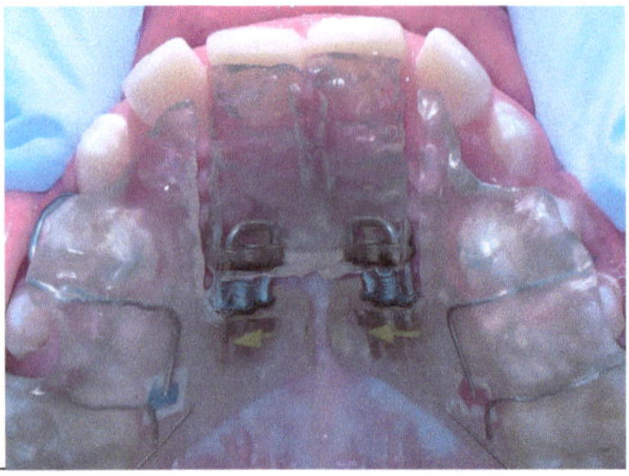
(G)

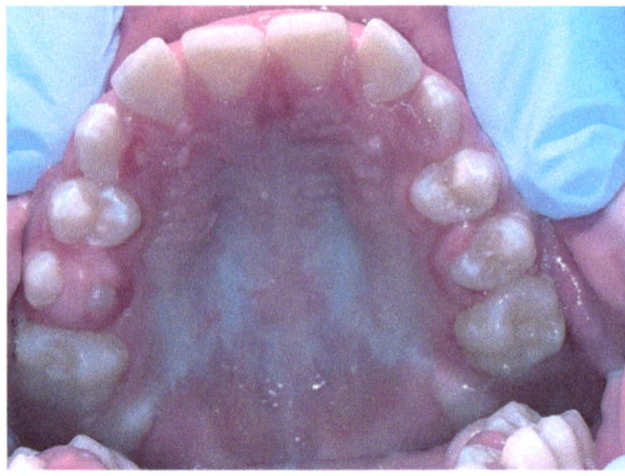
(H)

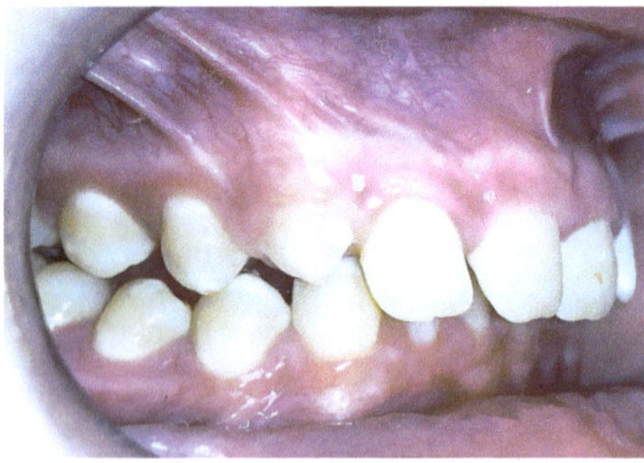
(I)

→ Figures 9-2 (G - I): After numerous months of wearing (and activating) the Sagittal II, the upper front teeth have been orthodontically cleared forward—moved "out of the way," so to speak, bone and all. This accommodated the subsequent *mandibular advancement* (or relocation) of the lower jaw. Compare Figure 9-2 (I) to Figure 9-2 (F) above. Note how, now that the deciduous cuspid (or baby tooth) has fallen out, the upper right permanent cuspid is now erupting into proper position.

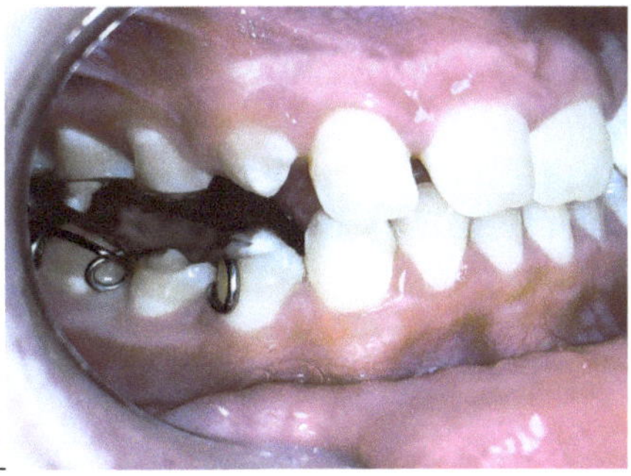

(J)

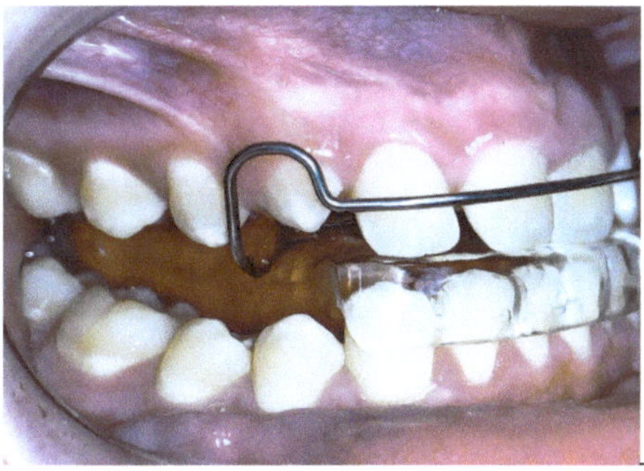

(K)

→ Figures 9-2 (J, K): These images show a daytime lower chewing splint as well as a special nighttime functional appliance called a Bionator. Following the Sagittal II, both were used to move the lower teeth, lower jaw, and the two temporomandibular joints forward, relocating them from their pre-treatment "dislocated" positions. What's really noteworthy here is that this young boy reported his migraine headaches were dramatically reduced after just the first two weeks of treatment. By the end of the first four weeks, he conveyed they had decreased by an astounding 90%! (Prior to the start of functional appliance treatment, the patient was prescribed harsh migraine-fighting adult drugs.)

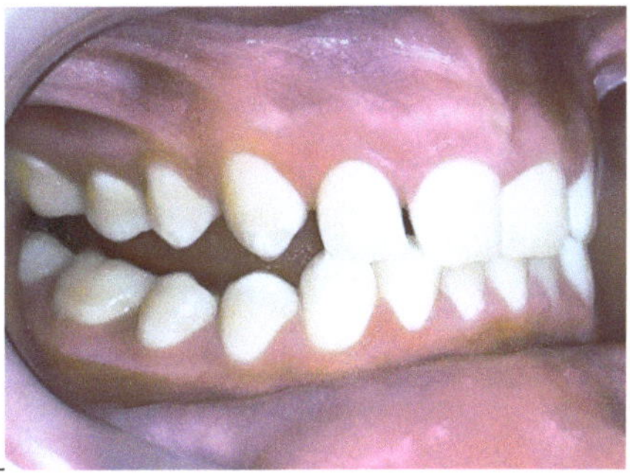

(L)

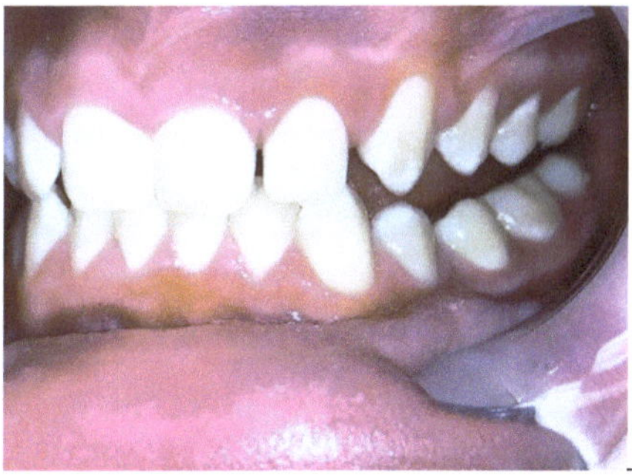

(M)

→ Figures 9-2 (L, M): You'll notice here the mandible has been fully advanced and healed to a down-and-forward corrected position, with the offending backward-tilted upper front teeth cleared forward, out of the way, to a correctly angulated position (this was accomplished by means of the preliminary removable active plate). In this relocated position, the now-healed lower jaw cannot be forcibly moved back to its former pre-treatment dislocated position. The mended TMJs won't allow it. (They won't allow the migraine headaches to return, either!)

(Continued)

Now, all that remains is to *verticalize* the back teeth toward one another, top to bottom, to complete the rebuilding of the bite. This is an easy and relatively quick orthodontic procedure, which uses modern orthodontic techniques that stem right from the FJO playbook of treatments. Dentists refer to this procedure as *closing a posterior open bite*. Posterior open bite closure—which pulls the back teeth together, top to bottom, in a permanently advanced or repositioned lower jaw—is a common part of the modern functional orthodontic/functional jaw orthopedic approach. Orthodontically, and orthopedically, it's a whole new, more-global methodology. (No harsh drugs are needed, either.)

Special Reader's Note: The principle of a *posterior open bite* can be easily demonstrated by a simple, little experiment. First, close down fully on all back teeth in your normal bite. Now, while keeping your teeth gently touching, slide your lower jaw forward, just a bit, so that your upper and lower front teeth touch (as though you are trying to bite off a piece of thread, or trying to tear open a plastic bag with your front teeth). Next, while holding the biting edges of your upper and lower front teeth together, stick your tongue sideways between what are now your (somewhat) vertically separated upper and lower back teeth. That little open space you feel between your top and bottom back teeth is a momentary posterior open bite. Because you have moved your lower jaw forward while keeping your upper and lower front teeth sliding against each other, this lower-jaw motion forces the entire mandible (and its passenger lower back teeth) to move downward. Hence, the appearance of that momentary posterior open bite.

Now, repeat the same experiment—only this time, don't slide your lower jaw quite as far forward. Once finished, use your tongue to feel how—with less forward movement of the jaw—the posterior open bite is correspondingly smaller. Simply put, less forward movement of the lower jaw equals less downward movement of that same jaw, which, in turn, equals a much smaller posterior open bite. Similarly, a more forward movement of the lower jaw means a more downward movement of that same jaw (and a greater posterior open bite). See how it works? Some dentists have a hard time accepting this relatively simple concept—especially as it pertains to orthodontic and/or TMD treatment—because they don't fully grasp the newer principles of mandibular (and hence condylar) advancement techniques. Which is unfortunate, as such modern methods can be absolutely critical for treating certain cases. Once the lower jaw, and its two sockets, have been put right and thus fit properly, handling an accompanying posterior open bite is no problem. You merely have to close the back teeth together vertically (using modern orthodontic techniques) until they hit correctly once more. That's it! Then just retain as normal. What could be better?

But if your child *does* have clicking, mild popping, or pain in their jaws during chewing—or if they possess a long history of worsening headaches (or migraines) that occur several times a week, over a period of months or years, without any other suitable medical explanation (or effective treatment)—

Here is what you must look for and insist upon:

- Ask if the plan proposed by the treating clinician is designed to allow—or even forcefully encourage—your child's lower jaw to come forward slightly (2–4 millimeters) in the fit of the teeth once treatment is complete. This should eliminate repeated, tension-type (somewhat milder) headaches and/or migraines.

- Ask the treating clinician if a radiograph might be obtained prior to beginning treatment. These films should be of each specific jaw joint, with the back teeth closed all the way, and not just as part of a larger general head or jaw X-ray. Such a film should show you how deep (proportionally) the lower jaw's condyles travel into each socket at full bite.

- After taking the radiograph, ask if there is any indication that either of the two mandibular condyles, right or left, are jammed too far back into the sockets at the teeth's full bite—and, if so, what needs to be done about it. Just because your child doesn't experience headaches, yet, doesn't mean TMD trouble isn't cooking just below the surface.

- Don't be afraid to ask additional questions or get another opinion. If you or your child have already had braces and are still suffering from TMD-induced clicking, joint pains, facial discomfort, and chronic, recurrent headaches, you're not "out of the picture" as far as getting it corrected. In fact, thanks to the orthodontic brace work you've already had completed, you're probably off to a good start.

Regarding that final point, you must realize you cannot—I repeat, *cannot*—blame your former orthodontist or general clinician for your current TMD problems. Many factors go into the development of such issues; it would be near impossible to prove your current TMD-headache condition was a result of the orthodontic treatment you received in the past. Chances are good that it wasn't.

At best, all you can really deduce is that, although you've already had braces and your teeth appear straighter on the surface, something still isn't quite right, namely the fit of your bite and the subsequent issues deep inside your jaw sockets (the presence of chronic, recurrent headaches and/or migraines bear the proof: Within the jaw joints, there's still an issue of misalignment). In which case, you probably just need your bite reset a little more forward, that last extra bit that will help clear the operation of the joints at full bite and restore the normal unpressured condyle-disc relationship.

People with recurring TMD-related problems who've already had braces can almost invariably be treated (quite easily) to a headache-free or very nearly headache-free state. Often, they're easier to treat than people who haven't yet had braces, simply because much of the preliminary "busy work" of straightening and properly aligning the individual teeth—as well as correctly shaping the upper and lower dental arches—has already been done. These types of patients turn out very nicely when the fit of the bite needs to be reset to correct a related jaw joint misalignment problem, especially in the hands of someone who knows what they're doing, TMD-wise.

Yes, it would have been nice if all of the work could have been done simultaneously the first time around. Yes, it would have been nice if those original braces had done the trick, or if those bicuspids (in some instances) hadn't been extracted, which just might've compounded the problem by shrinking back the bite. But knowledge is ever changing, and it's unrealistic to expect perfection on everything, especially the first time around. Just be glad we live in a time when the proper methods are now available, even if it does take an additional round of treatment in adult patients who've had prior orthodontics. Sometimes, that's just life.

The average orthodontist is a conscientious professional devoted to delivering top-notch orthodontic care to each and every patient. Orthodontists don't ever deliberately try to cause TMD problems; it's simply that this new knowledge is so vast in its scope—so revolutionary in its approach—that it'll take some time to filter down through the rank and file of average practitioners. And that's okay. At least the treatments are now available, bolstered by a brilliant track record of success and by plenty of hard-core scientific evidence affirming why they work.

The choice is now in your hands.

TEN

What About My Own Migraines?

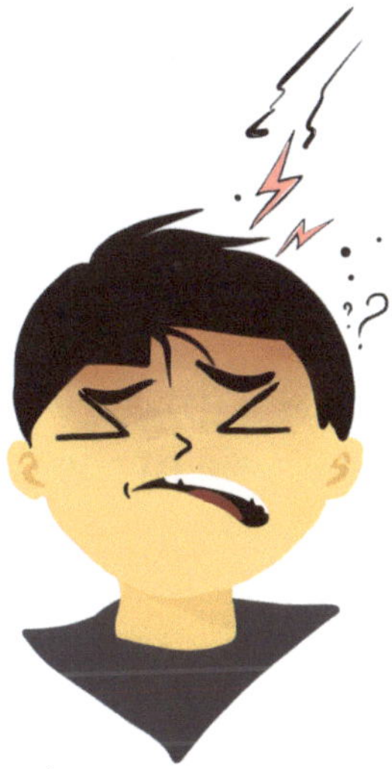

There is, however, a limit at which forbearance ceases to be a virtue.

— Edmund Burke (1729–1797), Irish statesman

Perhaps while journeying through this little book you've been thinking: "What about me? What about *my* recurring headaches/ migraines?"

Have no fear. We're about to explore this subject in depth, looking at—most notably—the more than 97% chance you have of experiencing either complete relief or an incredibly dramatic reduction in your nagging, long-term tension-type headaches and/ or migraines by means of the following advanced methods. Read carefully (but remember, nothing in healthcare can ever be 100% guaranteed—well ... except death!).

If you have chronic, recurrent headaches—be they the milder tension-type, the more sinister migraines, or a mixture of both—that have progressively worsened in frequency, intensity, duration, and are regularly accompanied by neckaches, the odds are likely that you have some form of TMD.

Let's look at some of the other potential symptoms:

- Your jaw joints "click" when you open and close your mouth.
- You once had jaw clicking, popping, or catching that bothered you when you were younger but, in the last several years, has seemed to lessen or disappear all by itself ... only to be replaced by a grating, squishy, or "rubbing-sandpaper-against-sandpaper" sensation upon movement and chewing, accompanied by a worsening of your headache problem.
- You have an occasional buzzing or ringing in your ears, or they feel stuffy or ache all by themselves.
- You get nauseated because of your headaches.
- You get extremely bothered by bright lights, loud noises, or certain smells during a headache attack (or those things precipitate a headache attack).
- Your jaws hurt when you chew gum too long or when you chew too many peanuts.

- Your headaches seem to throb and pulsate above or behind one or both eyes.
- You have headaches three, four, or five times a week (or every day), along with all of the above accompanying symptoms and a host of other head, jaw, teeth, ear, and neck pains that contribute to your overall headache problems.
- No otolaryngologist, neurologist, OB-GYN, internist, ophthalmologist, radiologist, chiropractor, or any other healthcare officer can find anything wrong with you that would otherwise be causing these symptoms.

Experiencing any, or all, of the symptoms listed above? Then guess what: The chances you're suffering from TMD are virtually 100%.

In fact, the relationship between TMD and long-term T-type headaches and/or migraines is so strong that, in the case of an adult, if the patient has had chronic, recurrent headaches for a year or longer, it's safe to assume the issue is a TMD one, until proven otherwise.

Migraines come from TMD syndrome; no other cause or mechanism has been discovered that's responsible for them. None! Don't be fooled by the so-called migraine "triggers." Certain things *do* prompt a migraine, but only in *migraineurs* (people who already suffer from chronic, recurrent migraines). A trigger is not a cause. So, what causes certain people to become migraineurs in the first place? For a child with chronic, recurrent headaches, one can almost invariably deduce (and declare) that the issue stems from a strained set of jaw joints—again, until proven otherwise.

(Another astounding discovery was recently made concerning problems arising from TMD. Certain types of rare muscle control movement disorders—possibly even the now-famous Tourette's Syndrome—appear to be related to the strained jaw joint condition of TMD.)

The TMD-headache connection represents one of the biggest breakthroughs in all of healthcare. *How so*? you may be wondering. Although the problems of chronic, recurrent headaches are not life-threatening, they certainly can be "quality of life" threatening, meaning they can drastically impede and disrupt the everyday lives of the condition's hapless victims. They number in the millions; just ask around.

How many people do you know who suffer from headaches several times a month—or even two, three, or four times a week? How many have migraines? How many have children with chronic, recurring headaches to the tune of one per month, or even once a week (or more)? How many have children who suffer from full-blown migraines? (Studies show 4% to 6% of all children under 12 do so.) With the exceptions of a cold, the flu, or other types of serious childhood diseases, no child should ever suffer from chronic, recurring headaches—*no* child. And don't be fooled by the old belief that if children get headaches above or behind their eyes, "Well then, maybe it's just because they need glasses." Maybe they do. When a child's eyes don't focus correctly or accommodate properly at certain distances, the child simply doesn't see well—which has nothing to do with repeated headache pain above or behind the eyes. Do deaf people get headaches simply because they don't hear well?

If you're an adult with chronic, recurrent headaches/migraines—as well as TMD-related jaw, neck, and shoulder pains—what, then, is the best solution for you? There always is the traditional choice: i.e., mask it all as much as possible with drugs and related *palliative* techniques. Sometimes, due to economic circumstances, that's all that can be done. If that's the case, fine, take the pills. It sure beats suffering all the time. But if you wish to attack the source, there are several modern treatment types you'll need to employ.

With TMD, your lower jaw is in the equivalent of a functional prison (driven back too far by your bite, by about 2–4 millimeters) and the jaw sockets are dislocated in a very sneaky way (though they are dislocated just the same). According to the laws of *orthopedic medicine* (the branch concerned with treating bones and joints): "If it comes in broken, put the two damaged parts back together and hold them there until they're as good as new again." Think of a broken arm or leg. The same "first commandment" of orthopedics also pertains to dislocated joints. If a patient comes in with a joint that's dislocated, primary treatment calls for relocating the separated parts back together again and keeping them there until the torn-up internal structures can heal themselves (as with a dislocated shoulder, knee, and, yes, even with slightly dislocated jaw joints). A joint is a joint is a joint: Whether for a knee, shoulder, or TMJ, the principle is the same.

Unfortunately, relocating a pair of dislocated jaw joints can get a bit complicated. You have to change the way the jaws chew, which means changing how the muscles close the jaws habitually as well as changing how the teeth fit when they chew. It's a tricky process. But, thanks to the modern techniques previously described, it *can* be done. And when done properly, the relief of TMD symptoms can be relatively quick—and quite dramatic.

To heal the internal joint damage and relieve the pain in the deteriorated jaw sockets, a series of special removable bite guards called *splints* must be worn. Some are used for chewing during the day; a second kind is used at night. The sleep-only variety often work best for the patient, but, because of their particular design and the way they fit in the mouth, they can't be used for chewing and eating during the day.

Like fishing lures, these individualized removable bite guards come in a range of shapes and sizes. They're handmade on plaster casts (or molds) of the patient's dental arches and constructed in such a way to allow the daytime chewing splint to snap onto the patient's lower arch of teeth. As the patient bites together, the acrylic intra-oral splint bites against the upper teeth, in a way that braces the movable lower jaw to a slightly more forward and correctly realigned position at full bite. This forces the condyles to seat themselves in a more proper location within their sockets, keeping those condyles from mashing the small sets of nerves and arteries in the upper back dome of the socket. Hence the splint "relocates" the dislocated condyles to their normal, pain-free operating position during chewing. It's a clever concept.

Some call these devices splints; others refer to them as "appliances" or *orthotics*. But for the patients who benefit from their immense relief, these devices are just plain wonderful! Although easily removable by either the patient or the dentist for hygiene purposes and other practical reasons, these snap-in bite guards should be worn day and night, especially during eating. Generally, they are used for about nine to 12 months, or until the jaw sockets are fully "hard healed." You can't stand on a recently healed broken leg, for example, until the damaged parts of the bone are fully knit together and strong once more. Otherwise, the fracture site will slowly start to come apart again under a workload. Same goes for human TMJs. And remember, internally damaged jaw sockets must heal "on the fly." Patients still need to chew, talk, and swallow. This makes the process different than that of a broken arm or leg in a cast. Even with the splints, the jaw joints are always moving.

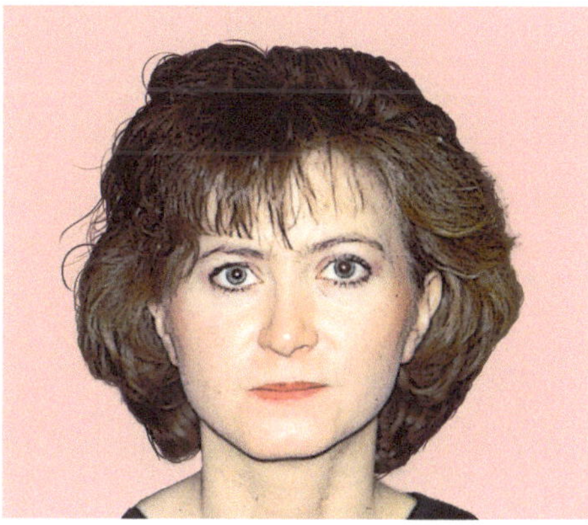

(A)

→ Figure 10-1 (A): This is a pre-treatment frontal view of a 29-year-old female patient who'd been suffering from terrible headaches for years. At the time of this photo, she was experiencing a particularly vicious type of end-stage migraine known as *status migrainosus*. These are terrible headaches! Most migraine headaches last between four and 72 hours; in status migrainosus, however, the attack can continue nonstop, without any let up, for weeks. This patient was suffering so greatly and so constantly that she was admitted to two different hospitals (in two different cities) and remained for about a week in each. Once admitted, she was bedridden while doctors treated her with powerful *intravenous* (IV) drugs. Sadly, she was then dismissed from both facilities after having been told they could do nothing more for her to help relieve her pain.

(Continued)

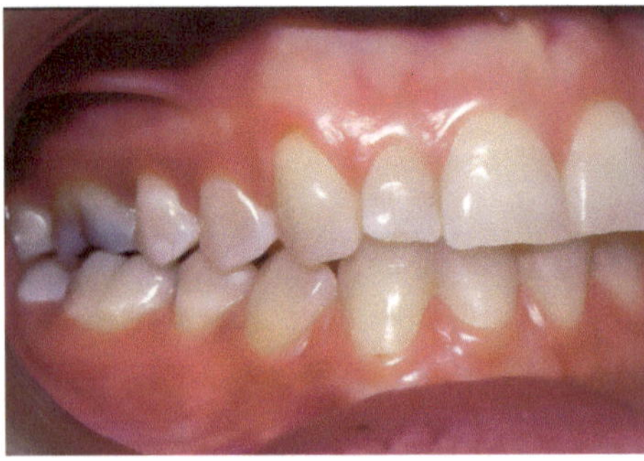

(B)

→ Figure 10-1 (B): An initial, superficial appraisal of her pre-treatment occlusion appeared fairly normal. Yet, X-ray-generated images of her TMJs at full bite revealed that both the right and the left jaw sockets were severely jammed by the "natural" fit of her teeth. Furthermore, the jaw bones themselves exhibited advanced bone damage and bony degeneration (known as *osteoarthritic regressive remodeling*).

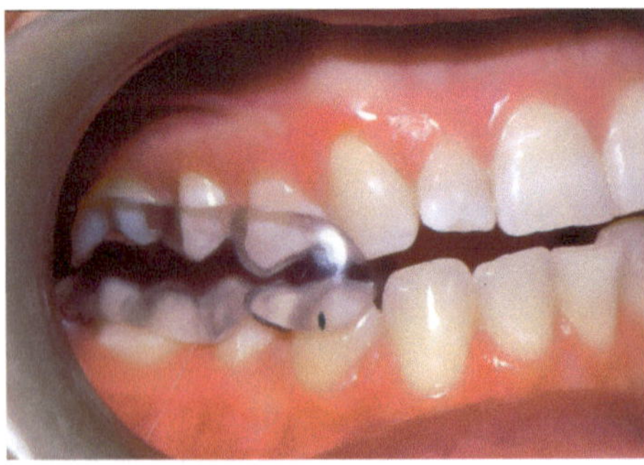

(C)

→ Figure 10-1 (C): This image shows a removable, X-ray-designed custom snap-on splint used for daytime chewing (i.e., a lower bite guard). You are viewing it from the right side as the patient bites down into it. This advanced type of splint is referred to as a FACT appliance, or a *functional advancing condylar translation* appliance. (It's easy to see why the term was shortened to FACT, but the acronym also serves as a timely reminder that it's a *fact* that this type of treatment works!) As previously stated, this splint is customized; it is constructed by hand, using X-ray measurements from the patient's jaw sockets, and is designed in such a way that, when the patient bites into it during chewing and/or swallowing, it forces the upper back teeth to interlock with its mechanisms while also causing the lower jaw to sit in its sockets in a properly relocated (or natural) way. All of which relieves pain.

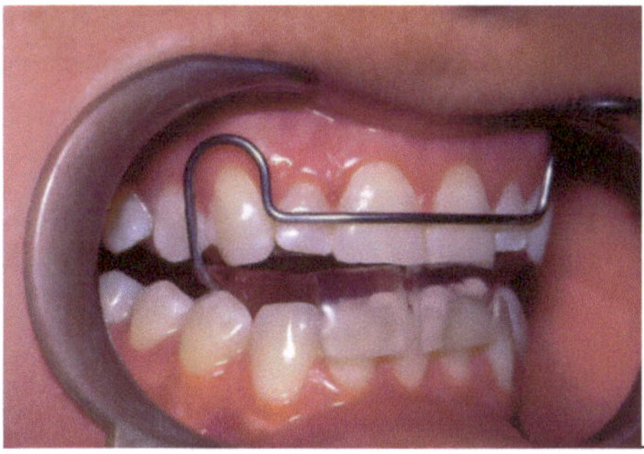

(D)

→ Figure 10-1 (D): A lateral view of the famous Bionator functional appliance, one of the world's best "muscle fixers." The patient wears it during sleep at night. Its use also has the positive side effect of helping the patient breath better during deep sleep. Which is also good! Note: The patient wears the removable FACT appliance throughout the day (and especially for eating). It's very comfortable and hardly shows; additionally, it doesn't bother the patient's speech. Following her day-to-day activities, the patient then removes the FACT appliance and inserts the Bionator for sleep.

(E)

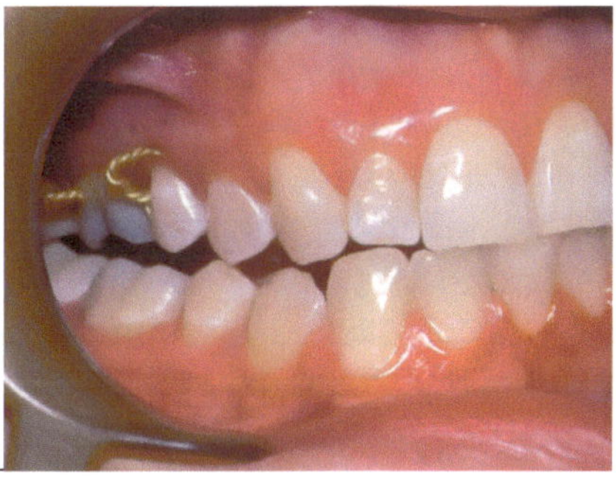

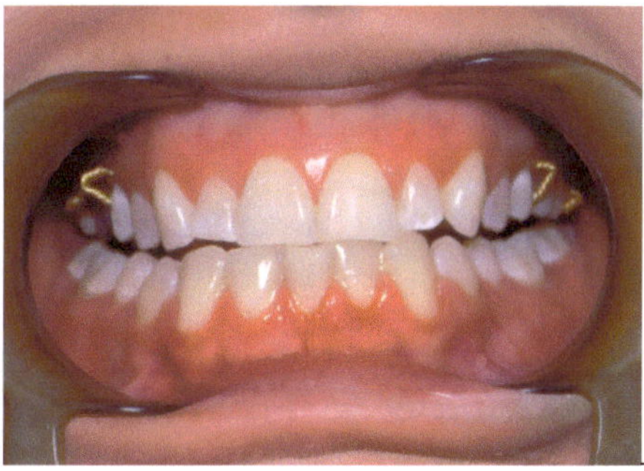

(F)

→ Figures 10-1 (E, F): Treatment for healing the patient's TMJs lasted about nine to 12 months. At the end of that period, the mandibular condyles had been relocated from their pre-treatment dislocated, pain-producing position. The case was now nearly finished.

During treatment, the entire lower jaw had been permanently repositioned (and healed) not only a little bit forward, but also a little bit downward. As a result, the lower jaw's passenger back teeth were also in a different vertical position relative to the upper back teeth (which hadn't changed). Because of how human jaws work, in this position, the lower jaw is now hard-pressed to close the gap between the upper and lower back teeth (posterior open bite). But that effort alone is counterproductive to pain-free joint operation: It's the equivalent of forcing the lower jaw (and socket) to go back to its original pain-producing position. Not good! Besides, such a process is nearly impossible with the lower jaw now healed in this advanced, corrected position—not to mention it would take many months for the jaw sockets to tear loose once the patient's appliance wear was prematurely terminated.

So, alternatively, the proper treatment at this point is to get the back teeth to fit properly *in conjunction* with the lower jaw's new, proper alignment. Case finishing then, in this instance, is predicated upon closing that little vertical gap between the upper and lower back teeth (*after* the lower jaw has been healed). *Not* fixing that gap—while at the same time taking away the appliances—would, as mentioned, result in the lower jaw slowly, but surely, dislocating itself and ripping its jaw sockets back to the original (painful) pre-treatment position. Again, not good! The headaches would return—and likely worse than ever.

At this point, the solution is to get each of the upper and lower back teeth to sit up a little higher in their sockets, so that they can then make contact with one another, top to bottom, in a full-biting, corrected jaw closure. This, in turn, would support the advanced lower jaw, allowing it to operate properly in its newly healed, slightly down and forward, pain-relieving position.

In other words, we need to close-up that posterior open bite in the back, while the front teeth continue touching (albeit at a slightly increased VDO). This can be easily (and relatively quickly) accomplished through several months of modern, highly advanced orthodontic techniques. Moreover, the kind of braces used for this only need to be placed on the upper and lower back teeth—i.e., no braces are needed on the front teeth. Patients like that!

While it's true that, during this phase of treatment (typically lasting a few months), patients will not be able to bite on their back teeth, it's really not as big of a problem as you may think. For example, ask children who lose their baby teeth and are still waiting for the replacement adult teeth to arrive. They chew just fine! In truth, patients hardly notice that they're no longer wearing the now-discarded daytime chewing splint. And, each day, those upper and lower back teeth incrementally move closer and closer together—all while at the correct down-and-forward lower jaw height.

Eventually, those teeth do finally come into full biting contact at the newly corrected jaw and socket position. This new position keeps the lower jaw-and-socket combination working at the proper height and at the proper degree of advancement. There's a word for it; it's called *natural.* (As one great TMJ expert once put it, "You have to put the teeth in a position to support that joint.") Once all of this is accomplished, the case is finished. (Note: There are several additional ways to close up a mid-treatment posterior open bite, other than just using orthodontics on those back teeth. None of them, however, require surgery.)

Once the case is finished, the jaw sockets are completely healed and relocated at full bite. Additionally, the jaw muscles themselves are fully healed and corrected. Thus, all things are finally working together the way Nature intended.

Look back on Figures 10-1 (E, F); a mid-treatment posterior open bite is clearly visible. Usually, the vertical gap in such situations is not great (only 2 to 4 millimeters). Note: In these photos, the little brass "twisty ties" between a few of those back teeth were placed several days before the metal braces were put on (at which time, the ties were removed). They are called *separators*, and there are several kinds. (See the "Special Reader's Note" on p. 136).

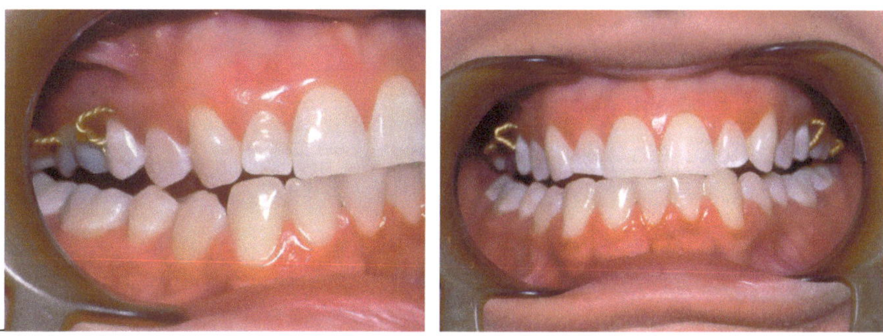

(E) (F)

→ Figures 10-1 (E, F): These images reveal now the patient's mid-treatment posterior open bite must be closed to full upper-to-lower back tooth contact. There, they will stay. The VDO will therefore be increased in conjunction with the mandibular advancement.

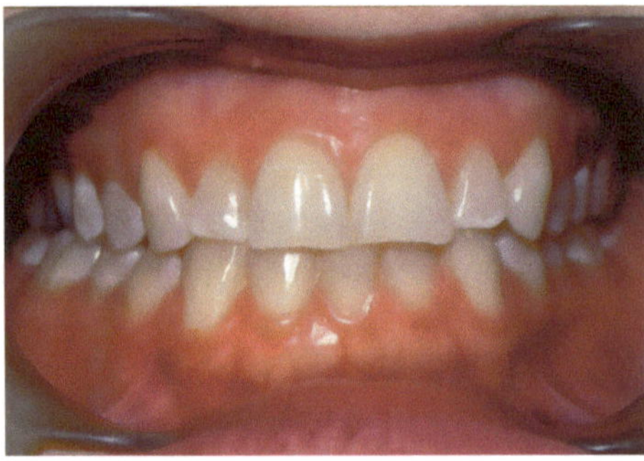

(G)

→ Figure 10-1 (G): This image is, again, the pre-treatment frontal view. Notice the VDO (the amount of overlap the upper front teeth possess over the lower front teeth at full bite).

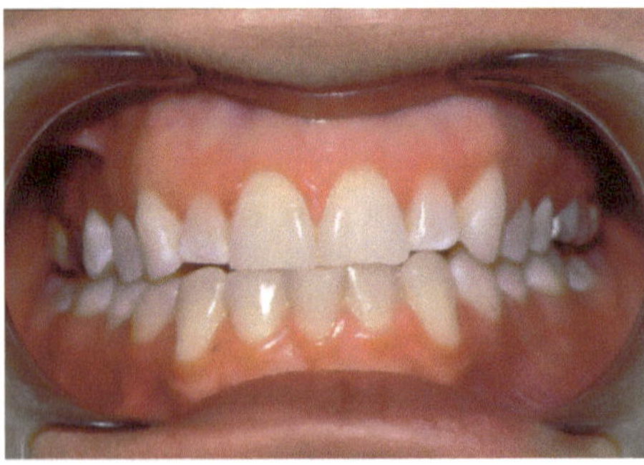

(H)

→ Figure 10-1 (H): A post-treatment frontal view. Look very carefully: The upper front teeth don't overlap the lower front teeth quite as much now. Observe the increased VDO, which is due to the lower back teeth now hitting sooner at full bite, as they are now higher in their respective sockets. This progress was the product of the posterior open bite closing techniques employed during the finishing portion of the mandibular advancement and relocation treatment plan. The distances involved in this approach may not, to the layperson, look like much, but, to Mother Nature, it's certainly enough. I'll return to an earlier analogy: How big is a grain of sand that you get in your eye? How does *that* feel? The spacing between the ball (condyle) and its socket (fossa) when they're closed together during the enormous power of full bite isn't substantial either. In other words, it doesn't take much anatomical misalignment while biting down fully to throw everything off—and, as a result, turn loose all of those jaw, facial, and headache pains.

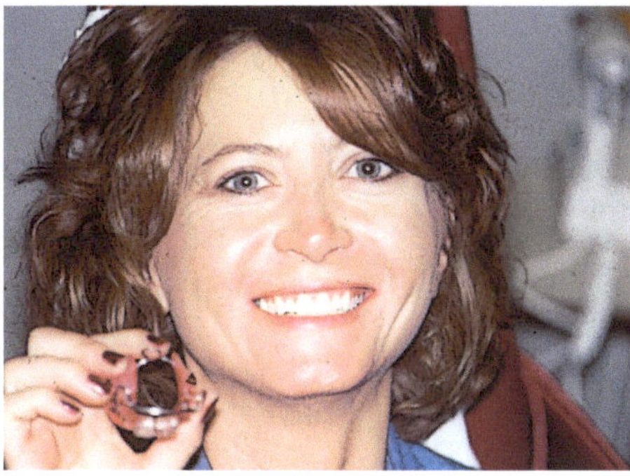

(I)

→ Figure 10-1 (I): The cured (happy!) patient shows off her final Bionator retainer, which was made to fit her new and improved post-treatment bite. She wears it only at night during sleep (and will do so for about a year after the completion of her treatment). And guess what: no migraines! They faded away over the first four to six weeks of treatment and, since then, have not returned.

Note: Remember: It's estimated there are approximately 27 million—yes, *million*—female migraine sufferers in America (an astounding number, and one that doesn't even take into account males). Likewise, 4–6% of all prepubertal children in America suffer merciless migraines, and that percentage goes up as those unfortunate children proceed to adolescence. We need to do something about this. After all, for about 99% of all migraine sufferers, we now have the cure!

The jaw joints finally "hard heal." With proper realignment and condylar repositioning treatments, headache/pain relief often reaches levels of 75% to 90% reduction within the first month—and even sometimes during the first week! Formal scientific studies show that within two months of the start of a splint treatment (known, in technical terms, as *anterior repositioning therapy*, or ART), 90% of patients were either completely headache free or very dramatically improved. And no drugs were used, mind you, just bite realignment with advanced types of TMJ splints. This is called *Phase I treatment*.

Of course, responses vary from patient to patient. Some take a little longer to recover than others. Total failure of correctly executed ART, however, is extremely—and I do mean extremely—rare.

There is only one problem that remains after nine to 12 months of splint treatment are completed and the patient is headache- and jaw pain-free. The upper and lower teeth will no longer individually match and fit, lowers to uppers, in quite the same way as their original full occlusion (or full biting) position. The lower jaw, which holds the lower teeth, has now been repositioned (correctly) to a slightly different and more advanced alignment position. To those dentists and TMD-treating clinicians who are used to doing things "the old way," the appearance of this slight but important permanent change (by means of intra-oral removable splints) appears really bad. For, when the patient closes his or her mouth with the splint out, the back teeth no longer come together all the way. As the slightly advanced lower jaw shuts, the upper and lower front teeth connect, acting as a "stop" that keeps the upper and lower back teeth somewhat apart. But, according to the new way of thinking, that's a good sign—one of success. It's very important to understand this. Here's why it matters.

When a bite is realigned forward (and the jaw joints are healed), the lower jaw automatically slides downward. In fact, you can't move the lower jaw forward *without* it descending to some extent. The lower teeth are one with the lower jaw; similarly, the lower jaw is one with its condyles. When you move the lower jaw—and hence its condyles—the passenger teeth inevitably move with it and will no longer align with the stationary upper teeth. For most patients, the accompanying downward movement is minimal, typically measuring 2–3 millimeters (though, for others, it can range as high as 5–6).

Thus, the problem is a little vertical gap that opens between the now more-forward bottom back teeth of the lower (repositioned) jaw and the stationary back teeth of the immovable upper jaw. In this state, the condyles can no longer jam back excessively into their sockets, as the back of each has filled in with properly healed tissues. The result: The entire lower jaw cannot move back as far as it used to, and the patient becomes headache-free. But there's still the matter of that little vertical gap, with only two clear solutions: 1) The patient must continue to wear the removable bite guards, splints, or appliances for life; or, 2) Something must be done to the now juxtaposed back teeth of the realigned lower jaw, ensuring they refit the upper back teeth and thus diminish/eliminate the gap.

But you can't just force those lower back teeth to fit into their original bite, as this would simply re-jam the condyles back into their starting places, too far back and up within their sockets, which, in turn, would re-smash all of that freshly healed soft tissue held inside, once more damaging the arteries and nerves and beginning the pain-headache process anew. Instead, you need to correct *both* problems: allowing the realigned lower jaw to close all the way in its corrected position while also verticalizing the back teeth (reapproximating their individual biting surfaces to make them taller, allowing them to once again hit properly during chewing in the new lower jaw position, without a splint).

Failing to do so is to invite disaster. For, without the protection of the splints, the lower jaw tries biting back too far, in an effort to get the rear teeth to connect. This gradually destroys the joints. Then the headaches and jaw pains return—and usually worse than ever!

(Okay, yes, there *are* certain exceptions. Technically speaking—on rare occasions—it is possible for a patient to have their lower jaw realigned more forward to prevent condylar jamming of the nerve bundle and then, after numerous pain- and headache-free months, the splints and functional appliances can be withdrawn, with the slightly advanced mandible allowed to gradually settle back to its pre-treatment retruded bite relationship, all without too serious of a relapse in symptoms. But such situations don't happen often, and, even if they do, the patient is still "on the bubble," TMD-wise. This type of hybrid technique [called a *walk-back*] is risky and, most of the time, fails. Upper and lower back teeth need to be verticalized once a lower jaw is healed in its more-forward and downward, corrected, headache-relieving position.)

There are only a few ways to verticalize the back teeth. You can:

- Provide the patient (adult or child) with orthodontics (braces) that will move the opposing back teeth together vertically.
- Perform cappings (also known as crowns) on a few of the adult patient's back teeth, making them "taller" and thus filling in that little vertical space while also allowing them to fit together in the newly realigned lower jaw position.
- Replace the original acrylic-based (plastic) removable splints with a more durable metal equivalent that, although removable, will last forever because it's made out of a special dental metal (it's called an *overlay removable partial denture*, or overlay RPD, and represents a more economical choice than the first two).

Once these finishing techniques are completed and stabilized, the patient is truly healed: no more headaches, migraines, jaw pains, or facial discomfort. The neck is usually a lot happier, too. I know what you're thinking: *Sounds too good to be true*. But make no mistake, it *is* true. It's merely a matter of what one famous researcher described as "... doing the right thing ... and doing the right thing, *right*."

Isn't that the secret to just about everything in life?

It's true these types of TMD treatments are a little involved, time consuming, and, at times, can be somewhat pricey, requiring a fair amount of commitment from both patients and doctors alike. As such, they're not for everyone. Yet they're by no means inordinately difficult or expensive either. And for those long-suffering migraine headache patients who truly need them, the relief they can offer seems like a miracle!

Now for one final hurdle: How do you find a dental clinician in your area who performs this kind of treatment? This step isn't always easy.

The best place to start is with your friendly neighborhood dentist. Ask the dentist if they provide these advanced treatment methods, and if they don't, ask if they can recommend a colleague who does. Many clinicians are now carefully studying (and using) these newer techniques, so the odds of finding the help you need grows every day.

Even so, while a number of dental clinicians now offer these types of orthodontic/TMD treatments, not every general dentist or specialist chooses to provide them. So, you'll have to be diligent in your research. Try calling your local or state dental society for help with a referral (or even just calling individual private practitioners).

Or you can start by contacting the offices of the International Association for Orthodontics (IAO), which is headquartered in Milwaukee, Wisconsin (www.iaortho.org). Check to see if one of their registered members practices near you (odds are good that if an individual is a member of the IAO, then the person has a command of many—or all—of the techniques previously described). Another possibility entails investigating the American Academy of Craniofacial Pain (AACP), which you can learn more about by visiting www.aacfp.org. Both groups are international organizations.

After reading this book, you now know what to ask for when calling a clinician's office. Ask if the doctor uses removable functional appliances of the European style when conducting orthodontic treatments. Find out if the doctor believes in them at all and recognizes the value of second molar extraction techniques in some selected cases for adolescents (or has even ever heard of it).

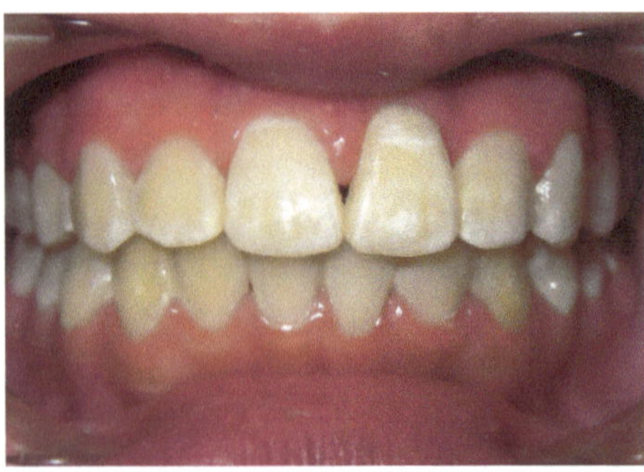

(A)

→ Figure 10-2 (A): In case you're interested—and by now, at this point in this little book, I'm sure that you are—here is an image showing how that first case pictured back in Figures I (A-C) turned out. These were taken at the completion of her treatment. Both traditional metal braces and functional appliances were used at various stages of the overall treatment process.

(Note: Some dentists might complain a little about the technical issue of the "midlines between the upper and lower front teeth being a bit off." To that, I say: So what? Look at how the midlines were positioned *before* treatment. Besides, the jaw joints are now perfect. That's what counts!)

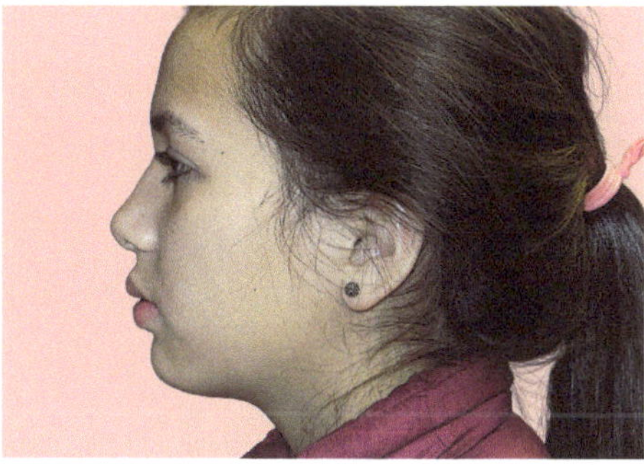

(B)

→ Figure 10-2 (B): Observe the post-treatment advanced profile of the lower jaw and chin. A sight to see!

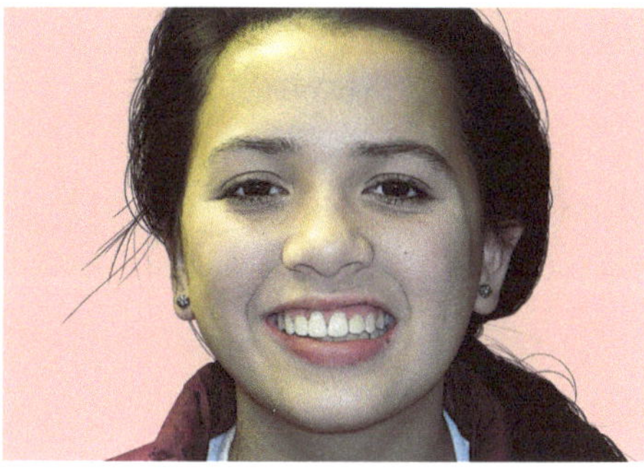

(C)

→ Figure 10-2 (C): A beautiful post-treatment result—and no headaches! Her jaw joint X-rays are perfect. Unlike in the beginning, the patient is now *delighted* to smile! Again, what could be better?

Ask—if seeking TMD treatments for yourself—if the doctor believes in permanently advancing the lower jaw just enough, in the final finished bite, to relieve TMD pains and related headaches. If the answer to any of these questions is yes, then you know you have an excellent chance of obtaining the finest in modern treatment techniques. Trust me, it's worth asking around.

(Which is why I put so much detail into this little book. I know at times it may have seemed like a tough read, but it was for your own good. Study these words carefully, so that you never forget what's best for your child's [or your] treatment needs. As far as the big picture is concerned, you now might think you know more in basic TMJ/TMD principles than some dentists. But don't get cocky; for, although this type of knowledge is empowering, if you tangle with a true professional, you'll be in over your head in no time! The devil is still in the details. And in this business, there are many.)

As a patient, you have every right to inquire. So don't get frustrated if the office you're calling gives you static—just blame it on me and this book! Fifty years from now this revolution in jaw realignment-style orthodontics for children (and related TMD treatments for adult migraines) will all be commonplace. Everybody will be doing it. For now, however, only certain clinicians provide it on a comprehensive scale, as such a massive departure from the status quo represents quite a methodological struggle. As you can imagine, there is a lot of money and ego involved. Even for yourself, all this information now swimming around in your head is probably unsettling, at least somewhat. I can assure you that the same is doubly true for many dentists.

On the other hand, there truly are numerous good, conscientious people in this business trying to help patients and families just like yours. A lot of them, in fact! As they say, it's better to light one little candle than to stumble around and curse the darkness. Remember, your average local dental clinician—be they a generalist or a specialist—really is a good person. So hope endures. The future is bright. And the wheels of progress are on the move.

For me personally, I've now finished my part in all of this. It was my duty to inform you, to ensure you have the tools, knowledge, and resources you need.

And now I have.

All that's left to say is ... good luck.

All we need to do is to voice these two petitions:
"Dear Lord, illumine my intellect to see the truth,
and then give me the strength to follow it."
It is a prayer that is always answered!

— *Most Reverend Fulton J. Sheen (1895–1979), American Catholic archbishop*

Bibliography

T. J.'s "Great Twenty-Eight" (Plus One)

Wisdom is much more important than knowledge.
There are a lot of fools with PhDs!

— Dr. Ben Carson (1951–),
American neurosurgeon and
2016 U.S. presidential candidate

When scientists argue over technical areas in their respective fields, one of the things they rely on to fortify their views is "the literature"—i.e., the articles, studies, and scientific findings published in authoritative journals. The most prestigious of these are overseen by a group of editors called *referees* (how appropriate). Their job is to read the papers submitted for publication and determine the validity/worthiness of each. It's not as straightforward as it sounds. Various fancy mathematical disciplines can get involved as well as classic principles of logic, experimental construct, and data manipulation. The goal is to preserve academic credibility and the widespread medical "canon," weeding out studies that exhibit bias or construct flaws. For example, in extremely complex subjects (like orthodontics), it is easy—if one has an agenda—to dig up some sort of study (or conduct an experiment in such a way) whose findings support just about any reasonable premise. That's what referees aim to prevent—at least in theory. But guess what: It doesn't always happen.

Take this example, for instance. Did you know—and this is absolutely true—that every single person who ate canned red tomatoes prior to 1865 is dead today? Must be due to something in those tomatoes, right? Wrong! Of course, you can immediately recognize the construct flaw in the logic behind the conclusion; it's obvious. But it's not always so apparent in more complex subjects found within science.

Even skilled referees can't always pick up on the flaws in complicated experiments, especially ones involving multiple topics in various-sized samples of individuals. There's an entirely separate discipline (with its own special rules) devoted to properly constructing valid studies in science. And there is an old—and rather harsh—expression that states: "Figures don't lie, but all liars figure!"

It seems inconceivable that educated scientists would be guilty of producing a so-called "study" that contains elements of bias. But it does sometimes happen, especially in areas as technically nebulous as healthcare. Usually such bias is innocent and merely a matter of the study's *experimenters* (or designers) selectively using the various bits of data they generate to support a preconceived notion. On complicated issues, it's an easy trap to fall into if you're not careful.

Generally, the literature in healthcare is pretty solid. If a study reflects, experimentally, what the clinician sees every day in their daily practice, then it's probably a good study. If it doesn't, further examination of the issue is required, until the truth of the matter is uncovered. Occasionally, researchers aren't convinced themselves of the validity of their findings. That's why, after summing up the conclusions of an article they're trying to publish, they'll sometimes hedge their scientific bets with statements like "But further studies are needed." And, truly, sometimes they are.

Another trick used by disagreeing scientists is the selective citing of literature. Like the notion of selective listening, individuals involved in highly contentious scientific debates will sometimes quote, study-wise, only what supports their agenda. And folks, we have to be honest here: The literature in the orthodontic/TMJ business is so vast, so varied, and (often) so difficult to keep in perspective, that if a person tries hard enough, they can find published materials to support just about any premise, no matter how ridiculous. (I'm being hyperbolic for effect, but I think you get the idea.)

Thus, below I present a brief, straightforward bibliography of what I consider ironclad, irreproachable studies from the orthodontic/TMJ literature that you can "take to the bank." Critics can rail all they want against what I say, but this list will stand firm against any argument, because, quite simply, this is the way it is. We're not playing games here; these findings mean business! Of course, there are many other excellent research articles out there, but for our purposes these will do.

(A note on formatting: This bibliography is summarized in the intervening paragraphs printed just below the related studies. These editorial analyses are written in academic language that's couched in fairly technical terms. I apologize, but these summaries are really meant to be read by dental professionals, to whom this bibliography is targeted. So, as a layperson, you can show it to your personal dental professional if you like, but don't get into an argument if the person seems disconcerted in any way. As I said before, you'd be in over your head in short order. But as a patient—or as the parent of a patient—you do have the right to ask questions, and you certainly have the right to the truth. That's only fair.)

Bibliography

1 .. Farrar, W.B.: Characteristics of the condylar path in internal derangements of the TMJ. J. Prosthet. Dent. 39: 319–323, 1978.

2 .. Weinberg, L.A.: Posterior bilateral displacement: Its diagnosis and treatment. J. Prosthet. Dent. 34: 195, 1975 (Part I). J. Prosthet. Dent. 36: 426, 1976.

3 .. Dolwick, M.F.: Normal and abnormal anatomy. In "Internal Derangements of the Temporomandibular Joints." C.A. Helms, R.W. Katzberg, and M.F. Dolich (eds.). Radiological Research and Education Foundation, San Francisco, 1983.

4 .. Eriksson, L. and Westesson, P.L.: Clinical and radiological study of patients with anterior disk displacement of the TMJ. Swed. Dent. J. 7: 55–64, 1983.

The above studies noted that internal derangements in the TMJs cause posterior displacements of the condyles at full occlusion, resulting in compression and injury to retrodiscal tissues of the highly innervated bilaminar zone.

5 .. Scapino, R.P.: Histopathology associated with malposition of the human temporomandibular joint disk. Oral Surg. Oral Med. Oral Path. Oral Radio. 55: 382–397, 1983.

In this study, Scapino histologically evaluated 17 TMJ discs that were surgically removed and described pathological changes in the disc and bilaminar zone due to the posterior condylar displacement of the disc.

6 .. Isberg, A.M. and Isacsson, G: Tissue reactions of the temporomandibular joint following retrusive guidance of the mandible. J. Craniomand. Prac. 4: 143–148, 1988.

In the above study, the authors placed composite and cast gold overlays on the teeth of monkeys that resulted in retrusive guidance of the mandible. After only five weeks, histological evaluation revealed thinning and flattening of the posterior band of the discs mentioned by Scapino above. They also observed inflammatory-type changes that occurred in the bilaminar zone similar to those described by Scapino.

7 .. Isacsson, G., Isberg, A.M. and Persson, A.: Loss of directional control of lower jaw movements in persons with internal derangements of the temporomandibular joint. Oral Surg. Oral Med. Oral Path. Oral Radio. 66: 8–12, 1988.

In this study, Isacsson studied the loss of conscious control of mandibular direction found in patients with internal derangements. 50 patients were instructed to move their mandibles laterally to an instructed position. 22 failed to do so properly. Of these, 18 out of 22 had proven internal disc displacement that did not reduce. The remaining four had internally deranged discs that did reduce. The loss of control was attributed to damaged mechanoreceptors injured by the posteriorly displaced condyles. When anterior condylar repositioning was performed, coordination returned in several of the patients.

8 .. Graber, T.M.: Temporomandibular joint disturbances and the periodontium. Int. J. Perio. Rest. Dent. 6: 33, 1984.

In the above publication, Dr. T.M. Graber, editor-in-chief of the

American Journal of Orthodontics and Dentofacial Orthopedics, states, "The condyle is brought forward in the fossa, and the neuromusculature may adapt to the new position, aided by occlusal interdigitation in habitual maximum contact, a new learned neuromuscular pattern or engram, and the filling in of a compressed retrodiscal pad, when it is no longer traumatized by the condyle."

Anderson, G.C., Schulte, J.K., and Goodkind, R.J.: Comparative
9 ·· study of two treatment methods for internal derangement of the
temporomandibular joint. J. Prosthet. Dent. 53: 392–397, 1985.

In this study, the authors divided 20 patients with internal derangements into two groups and treated them with either maxillary flat-plane splints (stabilization splints) or anterior repositioning splints (ARS). Those receiving ARS experienced significant reduction in the subjective and objective symptoms of the internal derangements. The patients who were treated with stabilization splints experienced no significant changes in dysfunction level. In fact, two of them worsened to a state of clinical closed lock!

Lundh, H., Westesson, P.L., Kopp, S., and Tillstrom, B.: Anterior
repositioning splints in the treatment of temporomandibular joints
10 ·· with reciprocal clicking. A comparison with flat occlusal splints
and an untreated control group. Oral Surg. Oral Med.
Oral Path. Oral Radio. 60: 131–136, 1985.

In this dramatic study, the authors evaluated 70 patients with internal derangements. Patients were divided into the ARS group, the flat–plane splint group, and an untreated control. Both splint groups had reduced joint tenderness, but the ARS group had greater reduction in the joint dysfunction and a greater decrease in muscle tenderness.

Williamson, E.H. and Sheffield, J.W.: The treatment of internal
11 ·· derangement of the temporomandibular joint: A survey of 300
cases. J. Craniomand. Prac. 5: 120–124, 1987.

In the above study, the authors evaluated 300 patients with internal derangements treated with anterior repositioning splints (ARS). After symptoms had been eliminated, the patients were switched to superior repositioning splints that guided the disc/condyle assembly back to the superior part of the fossa (i.e., only somewhat decompressed). Those who suffered relapses were given the choice of reinstating ARS or receiving arthroplasty. Three to five years after completion of treatment, patients were asked to grade themselves on pain, dysfunction, and remaining symptoms. Some 270 patients were still pain-free. Of the remaining 30 patients, 28 were initially pain free while being treated with anterior repositioning therapy. Their symptoms returned when ARS was discontinued.

12 .. Lundh, H., Westesson, P.L., Jisander S., and Erikson, L.: Disk-repositioning onlays in the treatment of temporomandibular joint disk displacement: Comparison with a flat occlusal splint and with no treatment. Oral Surg. Oral Med. Oral Path. Oral Radio. 66: 155–162, 1988.

In the above study, the authors evaluated 15 patients, one to seven years post-treatment. One group received disc-recapturing cast occlusal onlays. Another group received flat-plane occlusal (generic) splints. The third group served as a control. After six months, the group with anterior repositioning onlays (which had their mandibles correctly repositioned forward arthrographically) had significantly less pain and dysfunction than the other two groups. No significant difference was noted between the flat–plane splint group and the control. Most dramatically, once the onlays were removed, all symptoms returned within two months on all but one of the forward repositioned patients!

13 .. Lundh, H. and Westesson, P.L.: Long-term follow-up after occlusal treatment to correct abnormal temporomandibular joint disk position. Oral Surg. Oral Med. Oral Path. Oral Radio. 67: 2–10, 1989.

In the above study, the authors evaluated 15 patients one to seven years posttreatment. After an initial period of anterior repositioning therapy, which had subsequently been stabilized by means of either orthodontics or prosthodontics, 11 of 15 patients were evaluated with corrected sagittal tomography. Nine of the 11 patients had successfully maintained the therapeutic condyle-disc assembly relationship. Of the two who had not, neither were originally repositioned with the aid of arthrography. Yet, clinically, not one patient had pain either subjectively or upon joint palpation. This shows that some condyles can be allowed to settle or "walk back" as long as it occurs on a totally healed joint (healed by anterior repositioning therapy of sufficient duration). But it doesn't always work. In fact, more often than not, most walk backs fail.

14 .. Okeson, J.P.: Long-term treatment of disk interference disorders of the temporomandibular joint with anterior repositioning occlusal splints. J. Prosthet. Dent. 60: 611–615, 1988.

15 .. Farrar, W.B. and McCarty, W.L. Jr.: A Clinical Outline of TMJ Diagnosis and Treatment. 9th ed., Normandie Publications. Montgomery, Alabama, 1982.

16 .. McNiel, C.: The optimum temporomandibular joint condyle position in clinical practice. Int. J. Perio. Rest. Dent. 5: 71–72, 1985.

The above studies show that after successfully eliminating TMD headache pain dysfunction symptoms with anterior repositioning treatment, only about 25%–35% of the patients remained pain dysfunction-free after ARS was stopped and the mandible/condyle was allowed to settle back to its original pre-treatment occlusal position. Therefore, permanent anterior repositioning (relocation) is most often required. However, in certain circumstances, some modicum of "settling back" onto a well-healed joint is tolerated.

17 .. Blaustein, D.I. and Scapino, R.P.: Remodeling of the temporomandibular joint disk and posterior attachments in disk displacement specimens in relation to glycosaminoglycans content. Plast. Reconst. Surg. 78: 756–764, 1986.

This important study not only provides histological evidence for pseudo-disc formation after proper permanent anterior repositioning treatment of TMJ internal derangements, it also proves that many patients may be successfully finished "off the disc" in anterior repositioning therapy when disc deformity and/or other factors obviate disc recapture with ARS. Permanent decompression of the posterior joint space and its highly innervated bilaminar zone by forward/downward repositioning (permanently) of the condyle to the "Gelb 4/7 position" is all that is essential for relief of headache and joint pains. Disc recapture is a nicety but not a necessity. Getting the condyle advanced enough to decompress the bilaminar zone and keeping it there permanently in both rest and function, day and night, is a necessity.

18 .. Williamson, E.H. and Rosenzweig, B.J.: The treatment of temporomandibular disorders through repositioning splint therapy. J. Craniomand. Prac. 16: 222–225, 1998.

The above study is extremely important. It settles the TMD treatment issue once and for all in my mind. A sample of 160 patients treated for a whole host of traditional TMD headache pain dysfunction-type signs and symptoms—which were a result of posterior condylar displacement and internal derangement-type problems—were evaluated after anterior repositioning splint therapy. The average time for initial improvement was 22.3 days. The average time for complete remission of symptoms was 4.3 months. And here's the big one: Of all the patients, 89.4% experienced complete remission of symptoms and not a single one required surgical intervention.

19 .. Wexler, G.B., and Steed, P.A.: Psychological factors and temporomandibular outcomes. J. Craniomand. Prac. 16: 72–77, 1998.

This study, done by a master's-degree-holding TMJ specialist and a clinical psychologist on 561 patients, proves beyond any reasonable doubt that TMD signs and symptoms are not psychological in origin.

20 .. Grummons, D.: Orthodontics for the TMJ-TMD Patient. Wright and Co. Pub. 7819 E. Greenway Rd. Suite 5, Scottsdale, Arizona. 1994.

Additionally, here is an entire 351-page textbook—devoted to the treatment of TMD problems by means of orthodontics—written by an orthodontic specialist, with a number of its chapters written by other specialists the likes of Brenan Stack, R.M. Ricketts, A.H. Owen, and other equally prestigious clinicians, researchers, and experts. It states repeatedly that orthodontics is a correct and viable way to correct TMD headache pain dysfunction internal derangement problems. All told, there are hundreds of further references listed by these various authors that are associated with this concept.

21 ·· Brown, D.T. and Gaudet, E.L.: Temporomandibular disorder treatment: Second report of a large-scale prospective study. J. Craniomand. Prac. 20: 244–253, 2000.

In this study, the authors examined a whopping 2,104 treated, 250 untreated, and 44 long-term treated TMD patients using scientifically validated methods (the TMJ Scale to ensure uniform and valid assessment of treated outcomes) and concluded the following: "The use of anterior repositioning appliance therapy produced better results than flat-plane splint therapy."

22 ·· Simmons, H.C. and Gibbs, S.J.: Anterior repositioning appliance therapy for TMJ disorders: Specific symptoms relieved and relationship to disk status on MRI. J. Craniomand. Prac. 23: 89–99, 2005.

This university-based study clearly shows that chronic, recurrent headaches are the leading complaint of TMD patients, and 66% of a group of TMD patients were completely headache-free—and 33% rated themselves as vastly improved—after a course of mandibular anterior repositioning treatment. Some of the headache/TMD symptoms evaluated in this study were: pain behind the eyes, ear pain, tinnitus, TMJ arthralgia, clicking, and joint pain on chewing. Every single patient suffering from a lower jaw locking shut was relieved of that problem (i.e., a 100% success rate for that manifestation of TMD). The above cadre of symptoms also shows that both tension-type headaches and the more sinister vascular headaches (or migraines) are part of this scenario—thus, migraines can be initiated by TMD.

23 ·· Simmons, H.C.: White paper: Guidelines for anterior repositioning therapy for the management of craniofacial pain and TMD. J. Craniomand. Prac. 23: 300–306, 2005.

24 ·· Mintz, S.S.: Craniomandibular dysfunction in children and adolescents: A review. J. Craniomand. Prac. 11: 224–231, 1993.

25 ·· Schelhas, K.P., Pollei, S.R., and Wilkes, C.H.: Pediatric internal derangements of the temporomandibular joint: Effect on facial development. Am. J. Orthod. Dentofacial Orthop. 104: 51–59, 1993.

Ahn, S.J., Lee, S.P., and Nahm, D.S.: Relationship between tem-
26 poromandibular joint internal derangement and facial asymmetry
in women. Am. J. Orthod. Dentofacial Orthop. 128: 583–91, 2005.

The three studies above and "White Paper" produced by the American Academy of Craniofacial Pain conspire to produce a devastating cumulative effect. The white paper firmly attests that ARA (Anterior Repositioning Appliances—and that includes functional appliances) are the treatment of choice for TMD malocclusion-enhanced problems of anteriorly displaced discs that exist in concert with posteriorly displaced condyles, and that ARAs provide the best chance of displaced disc recapture via appropriate permanent mandibular advancement. The white paper was developed and approved by the AACP's own Board of Directors, a very erudite and prestigious group.

The Ahn, Lee, and Nahm study (as well as the Schelhas, et al. study published 13 years prior) shows that condyle-off-disc TMD problems can lead to facial asymmetries, stunted mandibular growth, and shortened ramal height on one side. If such problems occur unilaterally, a concomitant orthopedic distortion and facial asymmetry can occur. Not good!

The Mintz study is a survey of the literature from around the world that shows, on average, a minimum of 40% of all children presenting for orthodontic treatment already exhibit varying signs and/or symptoms of TMD. That's really not good (see Ahn, Lee, and Nahm above).

So, what this means in the real world is: 1) Examine for TMD; 2) If you find it, treat it—usually by means of some sort of ARA; and 3) If it's in a small child or adolescent, you'd better jump on it, the sooner the better. Facial distortions, unilaterally—as Ahn, Lee, and Nahm describe—or bilaterally, as could occur in Skeletal Class II retrusions, are only a harbinger of worse things to come if dysfunctional condyle-off-disc TMD is left untreated. Ask the chronic migraineurs.

Flores-Mir, C., Nebbe, B., Giseon H., and Major, P.W.: Longitudi-
27 nal study of temporomandibular joint disc status and craniofacial
growth. Am. J. Orthod. Dentofacial Orthop. 130: 324–330, 2006.

Here's a recent arrival that's just too important to pass over. In the above article, the authors show that when children and/or adolescents suffer from typical TMD symptoms—i.e., a condyle jammed too far back with its articular disc torn loose and displaced forward (referred to by these authors and researchers as "disc abnormality")—the entire jaw system suffers from a diminished and distorted growth of the bones. They concluded: "TMJ disc abnormality was associated with reduced forward growth of the maxillary and mandibular bodies. TMJ disc abnormality was associated with reduced downward growth of the mandibular ramus." So what this means is that not only does the lower jaw growth become distorted when a child or adolescent suffers from TMD (as 40% of them do, at least the ones that need braces; see the Mintz study above), but now it's even shown that the upper jaw (maxilla) suffers from reduced (distorted, improper) growth as well. Can the noose get any tighter?

Cooper, B.C., Kleinberg I.: Relationship of temporomandibular
28 disorders to muscle tension-type headaches and a neuromuscu-
lar orthosis approach to treatment. CRANIO. 27: 101–107, 2009.

Add to all this a more recent arrival: In this study, researchers show that the extensive literature (and their own clinical evidence) definitively supports the TMD-headache-migraine continuum. This study was performed—in conjunction with an extensive review of the literature—to determine whether there is significant evidence to support a relationship between headache and TMD prevalence. The authors state: "In the literature there was a substantial amount of evidence for positive relationship between TMD and prevalence of headaches and most importantly, that these were the muscle-tension type. The evidence for a cause and effect relationship was strong."

The authors further stated: "The benefits of resolving headaches at an early stage in their development is that it might result in the reduction of its potential for progress to a chronic and possibly migraine headache condition." These researchers were alluding to the TMD-headache-migraine continuum elucidated by other notable headache experts.

Yet despite all this, there are still those individuals who deny that the ortho TMD-headache-migraine connection exists at all. Such folks continue to claim there is no support for it. As the famous Italian astronomer Galileo Galilei once said, "It would not be enough even if the stars came down to earth to bring witness about themselves." (This was said as a reply to a letter from one of his students, Fr. Benedetto Castelli, concerning the rejection of certain astronomical discoveries by the hierarchy of the Church.)

The Plus One

Knowledge and beliefs regarding temporomandibular disorders among orthodontists. Am J Orthod. Dentofacial Orthopedics. 156: 4, 475-84, 2019.

And then there's this. They surveyed almost every orthodontic specialist in the country, 8,870 of them, by means of a questionnaire, about TMD (temporomandibular disorders, i.e., jaw socket problems). Only 1,545 of the orthodontists surveyed saw fit to answer the questionnaire (from their own people). The results were published in the October 2019 issue of The American Journal of Orthodontics and Dentofacial Orthopedics. It is by far the topmost formal and officially refereed orthodontic professional journal, published monthly in the United States. The authors of this article spent a good part of it grousing about how dentists used to mistakenly think that occlusion (fit of the bite) was a major factor in TMD, but that now, in these more modern times, "much wiser literature" says "not so much." (Bunk!) They now blame all sorts of other things, even psychological factors! But here's the big thing: The researchers conducting this massive survey found that almost 40% of practicing orthodontic specialists in the country, by their own admission, didn't "feel comfortable" in even just diagnosing TMD. Further, 50% of them confessed that they wouldn't even try to treat it, and a whopping 62% griped that they didn't feel "they received enough training in TMD during their orthodontic residency."

(Remember, in my fourth textbook, published in 2018, I explain and prove that chronic, recurrent, tension-type and/or migraine headaches are a TMD epiphenomenon that can be cured permanently by means of modern functional orthodontics.)

Question: Who's minding the store here?

Fere libentur homines id quod volunt credunt.
(Latin: “Most men are likely to believe what they wish.”)

— Julius Caesar (100-44 BC),
Roman general and emperor

About the Author

Terrance J. Spahl, Doctor of Dental Surgery, is a leading expert on orthodontics, maxillofacial orthopedics, and temporomandibular disorder (TMD). A graduate of the University of Minnesota, he has won numerous industry awards over an illustrious 50-year career, including "Clinician of the Year" by the American Association of Functional Orthodontics, the "Lifetime Achievement Award" by the Appliance Therapy Practitioners Association, the "Hayden-Stack Award" by the American Academy of Craniofacial Pain (their highest honor for a single recipient), and the esteemed "Leon Pinsker Award" by the International Association of Orthodontics (their highest individual award).

A certified Senior Instructor for the IAO, Dr. Spahl has lectured extensively on the subjects of orthodontics and TMD, lending his expertise to conferences across North and South America, Europe, Asia, and Australia. In addition to *The Headache-free Wonders of Functional Orthodontics*, he is the principal author of a quartet of textbooks, *The Clinical Management of Basic Maxillofacial Orthopedic Appliances, Volume I: Mechanics; Volume II: Diagnostics;* and *Volume III: Temporomandibular Joint,* as well as *The Clinical Management of the FJO/TMD/Migraine Continuum: An Evidence-Based Construct.*

Today, Dr. Spahl continues to lead the Spahl Dentistry practice in St. Paul, Minnesota, where he takes great joy in serving patients alongside his daughter, EmmaLee J. Spahl, DDS.

CPSIA information can be obtained
at www.ICGtesting.com
Printed in the USA
LVHW072053110421
683777LV00005B/1